CLINICAL EXERCISE SPECIALIST MANUAL

A FITNESS PROFESSIONAL'S GUIDE TO EXERCISE AND CHRONIC DISEASE

BY J. DANIEL MIKESKA, DHSC

ISBN-13: 978-1-946533-98-2
Published by Niche Pressworks; http://NichePressworks.com

Dedication

This book is dedicated to all of the educators who came before me, and to all of the educators who follow; may this book inspire you to never quit learning and to never quit teaching.

> If we could give every individual the right amount of nourishment and exercise, not too little and not too much, we would have found the safest way to health.
>
> Hippocrates

Exercise and activity are the best ways to address and prevent chronic disease. The succinct content combined with the easy to use tables and figures in this guide will benefit anyone who wants to learn more about any of the chronic diseases discussed, and how beginning an exercise program will improve quality of life.

This manual contains the most up-to-date information available at its printing. However, medicine and science are forever evolving, and newer information may have been distributed between the original writing and publication. Future editions will include any new, relevant science, and additional chronic diseases. Ideally, the concise information and format is to be used as a reference guide and not meant to be comprehensive. There are a number of educational programs or certifications that cover many of the topics addressed in this guide in much greater detail such as The American Association of Cardiovascular and Pulmonary Rehabilitation and the Cancer Exercise Training Institute.

The information in this manual is for educational purposes only and is not intended to be used to diagnose or treat any medical condition or disease. Anyone with a suspected disease or illness is encouraged to seek medical treatment from a licensed medical professional.

TABLE OF CONTENTS

Common Acronyms xv

INTRODUCTION TO CLINICAL EXERCISE: WHAT IS IT & WHY IS IT NEEDED? . . . XIX

Where We Are Today xix
Chronic Disease xx
Clinical Exercise xxi
Discussion and application xxii
References xxiii

CHAPTER 1—CHRONIC DISEASE AND THE BENEFITS OF EXERCISE 1

Chronic Disease Statistics 1
Common Terms 3
FITT 3
Clinical Exercise in the Healthcare Continuum 6
Discussion and application 6
References 7

CHAPTER 2—SCOPE OF PRACTICE AND HEALTH RISK 9

Scope of Practice 9
Pre-participation Screening 10
Par-Q vs. Physical Activity Risk Stratification 10
Health History 14
Informed Consent 14

Discussion and application 15
References 16

CHAPTER 3—RAPPORT AND PSYCHOLOGY. 17

Understanding Stress 18
Self-efficacy 18
Models of Behavior Change 19
Rapport 20
Educate Your Client 21
Be SMART. 21
Shaping 21
Discussion and application 22
References 23

CHAPTER 4—POSTURAL AND MOVEMENT ASSESSMENTS, & CORRECTIVE STRATEGIES. 25

Stability and Mobility. 25
Postural Distortions 27
Assessments 31
The overhead squat assessment. 31
Overhead squat assessment chart. 31
Overweight and obesity. 32
Discussion and application 34
References 35

CHAPTER 5—CARDIORESPIRATORY ASSESSMENT. 37

Definitions. 38
Maximal vs. Submaximal 38
Termination of Assessment 38
Metrics. 39
Ventilatory threshold. 39
Rating of perceived exertion and talk test. 39
EPOC 40
Discussion and application 40
References 41

CHAPTER 6—FITT 43

Aerobic Exercise 44
Muscular Fitness. 44

Flexibility 45
Neuromuscular Fitness 47
FITT guidelines 48
Discussion and application 49
References 50

CHAPTER 7—CORONARY HEART DISEASE 53

Background 53
Pre-participation Health Screening 54
Contraindications 55
Exercise Recommendations 56
Nutrition Basics 56
Discussion and application 57
References 58

CHAPTER 8—HYPERTENSION 59

Characteristics 59
Pharmacological Therapy 60
Exercise Training 61
FITT recommendations for hypertension 61
Caution 62
Nutritional Considerations 62
Discussion and application 63
References 64

CHAPTER 9—COPD AND ASTHMA 65

Chronic Obstructive Pulmonary Disorder 65
Statistics 66
Pharmacology and Nutrition 66
Activity 67
FITT guidelines for pulmonary dysfunction 68
Discussion and application 69
References 70

CHAPTER 10—DIABETES 71

Background 71
Diagnostic Criteria 72

Treatment Strategies 72
Exercise 72
FITT guidelines for diabetes 73
Exercise and Medications 73
Dietary Considerations 75
Complications and Concerns 76
Discussion and application 77
References 78

CHAPTER 11—HYPERLIPIDEMIA 79

Cholesterol and Triglycerides 79
Exercise 81
FITT guidelines for clients with blood lipid disorders 82
Nutrition 82
Medication 83
Discussion and application 83
References 84

CHAPTER 12—BODY COMPOSITION, OVERWEIGHT AND OBESITY 85

Statistics 86
Body Composition Metrics 86
Thermal Activity and Metabolism 88
Weight Loss and Dietary Guidelines 88
Pharmacology and Surgery 89
Exercise 89
FITT recommendations for overweight and obese 90
Discussion and application 91
References 92

CHAPTER 13—METABOLIC SYNDROME 95

Characteristics 95
Treatment Strategies 96
Nutrition 96
Pharmacology and surgery 97
Activity 97
FITT guidelines for metabolic syndrome 98
Discussion and application 98
References 99

CHAPTER 14—CANCER 101

Pathophysiology 102
Classification 102
Pharmacology....102
Lymphedema 103
Cancer Related Fatigue 103
Comorbidities 104
Modifiable Factors 104
Nutrition 105
Physical Activity 106
FITT guidelines for cancer prevention, treatment, and recovery 106
Considerations 107
Discussion and application 107
References 108

CHAPTER 15—PREGNANCY....111

Benefits of Exercise....111
Weight Gain Recommendations 112
Musculoskeletal Response 112
Physiological Response 113
Preeclampsia....113
Gestational Diabetes....114
Diastasis Recti 114
Precautions and Considerations for Exercise 114
Exercise recommendations for pregnant women....116
Postpartum Exercise Recommendations....116
Discussion and application 117
References 118

CHAPTER 16—CORE, BALANCE, AND GAIT 119

Movement and Stability 119
Postural Control....120
The Core 120
The Gait Cycle 121
Exercise Strategies....122
Core and myofascial sling exercises....123
Discussion and application 124
References 125

CHAPTER 17—COMMON SHOULDER DYSFUNCTIONS 127

Shoulder Anatomy 127
Scapular Dyskinesis 129
Exercise recommendations for scapular dyskinesis 130
Shoulder Pathologies. 130
Shoulder separation. 130
Shoulder impingement 131
Subacromial bursitis 131
Shoulder instability. 131
Interventions 132
Recommended exercises for shoulder sprain and instability, and rotator cuff injuries . . . 132
Discussion and application 133
References 134

CHAPTER 18—COMMON DYSFUNCTIONS OF THE DISTAL ARM 135

Anatomy 135
Epicondylitis 136
Carpal Tunnel Syndrome 137
De Quervain's Tenosynovitis 138
Recommended restorative exercises for distal arm dysfunction 138
Discussion and application 139
References 140

CHAPTER 19—COMMON HIP DYSFUNCTIONS. 141

Anatomy 141
Gluteal Trochanteric Pain Syndrome and Trochanter Bursitis 142
Iliotibial Band Friction Syndrome. 143
Osteoarthritis 144
Hip Replacement 145
Piriformis Syndrome. 145
Restorative exercise recommendations for common hip injuries 147
Discussion and application 148
References 149

CHAPTER 20—COMMON KNEE DYSFUNCTIONS 151

Anatomy 151
Patellofemoral Pain Syndrome. 153
Q-angle 153
Meniscus Injuries 154

ACL Injuries. 156
Total Knee Replacement 157
General activity guidelines for common knee dysfunctions 157
Discussion and application 158
References 159

CHAPTER 21—COMMON DYSFUNCTIONS OF THE LOWER EXTREMITY 161

Anatomy 162
Shin Splints 163
Ankle Sprains 164
Achilles Tendinopathy. 165
Plantar Fasciitis 166
General activity guidelines for common injuries of the lower leg, ankle, and foot 168
Discussion and application 169
References 170

CHAPTER 22—LOW BACK PAIN 171

The Prevalence of Low Back Pain. 171
Treatment Protocols 173
Education 173
Pharmacology and surgery. 174
Exercise. 174
Example exercises for low back pain. 177
Discussion and application 177
References 178

CHAPTER 23—ARTHRITIS 179

Background 179
Osteoarthritis 180
Pharmacology 181
Nutritional supplements 181
Exercise intervention 182
Rheumatoid Arthritis 183
Pharmacology 183
Nutrition 184
Exercise intervention 185
FITT recommendations for OA 186
FITT recommendations for RA. 186
Discussion and application 187
References 188

CHAPTER 24—OSTEOPOROSIS 189

Background 189
Statistics 190
Formation of Bone 190
Factors That Effect Bone Mass Density 190
The Female Triad 192
Pharmacology 193
Nutrition 193
Exercise and Activity 195
FITT recommendations for clients with osteopenia or osteoporosis 196
Discussion and application 197
References 198

CHAPTER 25—BUSINESS CONSIDERATIONS 201

Business Entities 201
The Health Insurance Portability and Accountability Act 203
Social Media 204
SOAP Notes 205
Ethical Considerations 205
Discussion and application 207
References 208

APPENDICES 209

Appendix A—Sample Physical Activity Risk Stratification form 210
Appendix B—Sample Medical Clearance form 212
Appendix C—YMCA Bench Step Assessment for Cardiovascular Fitness 213
Appendix D—Sample SOAP Notes form 214

Table 1 lists common acronyms used by fitness professionals and in this textbook.

Table 1

Common acronyms

1RM	One repetitions maximum
A1C	Glycated hemoglobin blood test for Type 2 diabetes and prediabetes
AC	Acromioclavicular
ACE	American Council on Exercise
ACL	Anterior cruciate ligament
ACOG	American College of Obstetricians and Gynecologists
ACSM	American College of Sports Medicine
ADL	Activity of daily living
ADR	Abdominal diastasis recti
ASCVD	Atherosclerotic cardiovascular disease
AT	Achilles tendon
ATFL	Anterior talofibular
ATP	Adenosine triphosphate
BMD	Bone mass density
BMI	Body mass index
BOS	Base of support
BP	Blood Pressure
CDC	Centers for Disease Control and Prevention
CFL	Calcaneofibular
CHD	Coronary heart disease
CKC	Closed kinetic chain
CO2	Carbon dioxide
COG	Center of gravity
COPD	Chronic obstructive pulmonary disorder
CPT	Certified personal trainer
CRF	Cancer related fatigue
CXS	Clinical Exercise Specialist
CTS	Carpal tunnel syndrome
CV	Cardiovascular
CVD	Cardiovascular disease
DBP	Diastolic blood pressure
DCER	Dynamic constant external resistance
DEXA	Dual-energy X-ray absorptiometry
DMARDs	Disease-modifying antirheumatic drugs
DNA	Deoxyribonucleic acid
DRI	Dietary reference intake
DS	Dynamic stretch
DXA	Dual-energy X-ray absorptiometry
EIB	Exercise-induced bronchospasms

EIM	Exercise is Medicine
EPOC	Excess post-exercise oxygen consumption
ER	External rotation
FFM	Fat free mass
FITT	Frequency, Intensity, Time, Type
FMS	Functional movement screen
GDM	Gestational diabetes mellitus
GH	Glenohumeral
GTPS	Greater trochanter pain syndrome
HDL	High-density lipoprotein
HHR	Heart rate reserve
HIIT	High intensity interval training
HIPAA	Health Insurance Portability Accountability Act
HIT	High intensity training
HR	Heart rate
HTN	Hypertension
IR	Internal rotation
IT Band	Iliotibial band
ITBFS	Iliotibial band friction syndrome
KSA	Knowledge, skills, and abilities
Lat(s)	Latissimus Dorsi
LBP	Low back pain
LDL	Low-density lipoprotein
LLC	Limited Liability Company
M/B	Medicine ball
MetS	Metabolic syndrome
MI	Myocardial infarction
MTSS	Medial tibial stress syndrome
NEAT	Non-exercise thermogenesis
NO	Nitric oxide
NSIADS	Non-steroidal anti-inflammatory
O/B	On ball
OA	Osteoarthritis
OHS	Overhead squat assessment
OKC	Open kinetic chain
OTC	Over the counter
PAR-Q	Pre-activity readiness questionnaire
Par-Q+	Pre-activity readiness questionnaire for everyone
Peak VO2	The highest value of VO2 attained upon an exercise test
PF	Plantar fasciitis
PFPS	Patellofemoral pain syndrome
PNF	Proprioceptive neuromuscular facilitation
RA	Rheumatoid arthritis

RD	Registered dietician
RICE	Rest, Ice, Compression, Elevation
RMR	Resting metabolic rate
RNA	Ribonucleic acid
ROM	Range of motion
RPE	Rating of perceived exertion
S/L	Single leg
SBP	Systolic blood pressure
SD	Scapular dyskinesis
SLR	Straight leg raise
SMR	Self-myofascial release
SOAP	Subjective, Objective, Assessment, Plan
SS	Static stretch
T1DM	Type 1 diabetes mellitus
T2DM	Type 2 diabetes mellitus
TEA	Thermal effect of activity
TEE	Total energy expenditure
TEF	Thermal effect of food
TEM	Thermal effect of metabolism,
THA	Total hip arthroplasty
TNM	Tumor, node, metastasis
TT	Talk test
VMO	Vastus medialis oblique
VO2max	Maximal oxygen uptake or maximal aerobic capacity
VO2R (reserve)	The difference between VO_2max and VO_2 at rest
VT1	First ventilatory threshold, also lactate threshold or anaerobic threshold
VT2	Second ventilatory threshold or respiratory compensation threshold

INTRODUCTION TO CLINICAL EXERCISE: WHAT IS IT & WHY IS IT NEEDED?

Where We Are Today

- In the United States, adults have decreased their number of steps per day by an estimated 70% since the Industrial Revolution (Booth, Roberts, & Laye, 2012)
- Screen time is estimated to be 7.5 hours per day for children and adolescents, adding up to over 114 days (Centers for Disease Control and Prevention [CDC], 2018).
- Time in front of the television has increased by 1% per year for the past 50 years to a current median time of 4.5 hours per day (Brownson, Boehmer, & Luke, 2005; CDC, 2018)
- More screen time is associated with (Twenge & Campbell, 2018):
    - o Lower psychological well-being
    - o Less curiosity
    - o Lower self-control
    - o More distractibility
    - o More difficulty making friends
    - o Less emotional stability
    - o Being more difficult to care for
    - o Inability to finish tasks

- The average adult spends only 1%-5% of each day performing moderate-to-vigorous activity (Hamilton, Healy, Dunstan, Zderic, & Owen, 2008)
- Less than 23% of U.S. adults, aged 18-65, meet the recommendations for aerobic and muscle-strengthening exercise (Waters & Graf, 2018)

Chronic Disease

Chronic disease is slow in its progress and long in its continuance, as opposed to acute disease, characterized by a swift onset and short course (Booth et al., 2012; Pedersen & Saltin, 2015; Spivey, 2015). Table 2 lists some examples of chronic diseases.

Table 2

Chronic diseases

• Low cardiorespiratory fitness (VO2max)	• Arterial dyslipidemia
• Asthma	• Hemostasis
• Sarcopenia	• Deep vein thrombosis
• Metabolic syndrome	• Cognitive dysfunction
• Obesity	• Depression and anxiety
• Insulin resistance	• Osteoporosis, osteopenia, and osteoarthritis
• Pre-diabetes, type I diabetes, and type II diabetes	• Balance disorders/falls
• Cardiovascular disease	• Bone fractures
• Peripheral artery disease	• Rheumatoid arthritis and other autoimmune disorders
• Pre-hypertension and hypertension	• Various forms of cancer
• Stroke	• And some conditions brought about by pregnancy
• Endothelial dysfunction	

Booth et al., 2012; Pedersen & Saltin, 2015; Spivey, 2015

Newton's third law of motion states for every action, there is an equal and opposite reaction. The reaction to the sedentary lifestyle adopted by a majority of U.S. adults is an overweight and obesity rate of over 70% (The National Institute of Diabetes and Digestive and Kidney Diseases, 2017). More than 63 million U.S. adults complain of joint pain, and by conservative estimates, close to 60% of individuals over age of 60 have some form of arthritis, as do one-third of individuals between the ages of 18-64 (Arthritis Foundation, n.d; Weinstein, Yelin, & Watkins-Castillo, 2015). Close to 50% of the population has at least one chronic disease, and the rate of comorbidities is rising. In adults under age 65, 25% have multiple comorbidities, and by 2030, there will be 70 million people age 65 years and over; and almost 75% will have multiple chronic diseases or conditions (Tinetti, Fried, & Boyd, 2012). Interestingly, at the same time lifespans have increased from about 70 years of age in 1970 to almost 79 years now. However, due to lifestyle shifts, poor nutrition, and increased inactivity, chronic disease now afflict the population at a younger age, meaning we will have to live with chronic diseases or conditions for a longer time.

The combined result is an unhealthy and aging population, placing undue financial burdens on society, and taxing an already strained health care system. Almost 70% of deaths in the U.S. are attributed to chronic disease, with an associated annual cost of almost $3.7 trillion in medical expenses and lost productivity. Over $1.4 trillion is attributed to cardiovascular disease, and obesity, which is by far considered the greatest burden, costs $1.72 trillion annually (American Public Health Association, 2014; Waters & Graf, 2018).

Clinical Exercise

Physical activity, defined as any bodily movement produced by voluntarily contracting skeletal muscle that results in energy expenditure above a basal level, can positively affect over 30 chronic conditions, making it the best deterrent of chronic disease in primary and secondary prevention. Therefore, the main goal of clinical exercise in the healthcare continuum is to prevent the onset of chronic disease. (Ali & Katz, 2015; Booth et al., 2012; Durstine, Gordon, Wang, & Luo, 2013; Spivey, 2015).

Clinical exercise helps bridge the gap between clinical intervention and conventional fitness programs (Muth, 2007; Williamson, 2010). A clinical exercise specialist (CXS) develops exercise programs for individuals or groups that have, or are at risk for, chronic disease or dysfunction, or for individuals who need specialized care (Jacobs, 2018; Spivey, 2015). A CXS can work with clients and groups at risk for chronic disease, have health conditions that may be mitigated or managed by exercise and activity, are newly diagnosed with disease and need exercise guidance, or have completed a medically supervised rehabilitation program, such as cardiovascular or orthopedic, and need to continue to progress.

The Exercise is Medicine (EIM) initiative was established in 2007 as a collaboration between the American Medical Association and the American College of Sports Medicine. The main goal of EIM is to advance physical activity as a method of primary prevention in healthcare, and to encourage physicians to prescribe evidence-based exercise as an intervention in the management of chronic disease. Through interprofessional collaboration, EIM establishes referral networks and clinical teams to compliment and leverage the strengths of each team member to improve population health (Lobelo, Stoutenberg, & Hutber, 2014).

According to the World Health Organization (2010), interprofessional collaboration occurs when multiple health workers from different professional backgrounds work together with patients, families, caregivers, and communities to deliver the highest quality of care. Based on the growing incidence of chronic disease and comorbidities, it makes sense to manage the associated complex health care demands, using a team of providers with varying skill sets to collaborate and deliver the best care possible (van Dongen et al., 2016).

The role of the fitness professional is to work with a client's team of other healthcare providers. Building this medical network indicates a fitness professional's main goal is the wellbeing of a client. The team of providers may include:

- A nutritionist or registered dietitian
- A rehabilitation specialist or physical therapist
- A massage therapist
- A chiropractor
- A mind and body specialist such as Yoga, Tai Chi, or meditation
- A clients' referring physician who is the center of a client's healthcare team, and should be provided regular updates as to a client's progress (Mikeska, 2015; Spivey, 2015)

Discussion and application

1. What is Interprofessional Collaboration and how will it benefit your clients and your business?
2. What are some of the common deficits caused by inactivity, which ones have you experienced in your business, and how have you addressed them?
3. How would you define and describe Medical Exercise?

References

Ali, A., & Katz, D. L. (2015). Disease prevention and health promotion: How integrative medicine fits. *American Journal of Preventive Medicine, 49(*5 Suppl 3), S230-240. https://doi.org/10.1016/j.amepre.2015.07.019

American College of Sports Medicine. (2018). *ACSM's resources for the exercise physiologist: A practical guide for the health fitness professional* (P. Magyari, R. Lite, M. W. Kilpatrick, & J. E. Schoffstall Eds. 2 ed.). Philadelphia, PA: Wolters Kluwer.

American Public Health Association. (2014). Public health and chronic disease cost savings and return on investment. Retrieved from https://www.apha.org/~/media/files/pdf/fact%20sheets/chronicdiseasefact_final.ashx

Arthritis Foundation. (n.d.). Arthritis by the numbers: Book of trusted facts and figures. Retrieved from https://www.arthritis.org/Documents/Sections/About-Arthritis/arthritis-facts-stats-figures.pdf

Booth, F. W., Roberts, C. K., & Laye, M. J. (2012). Lack of exercise is a major cause of chronic diseases. *Comprehensive Physiology, 2*(2), 1143-1211. https://doi.org/10.1002/cphy.c110025

Brownson, R. C., Boehmer, T. K., & Luke, D. A. (2005). Declining rates of physical activity in the United States: What are the contributors? *Annual Review of Public Health, 26*, 421-443. https://doi.org/10.1146/annurev.publhealth.26.021304.144437

Centers for Disease Control and Prevention. (2018). About screen time. Retrieved from https://www.cdc.gov/nccdphp/dnpao/multimedia/infographics/getmoving.html

Durstine, J. L., Gordon, B., Wang, Z., & Luo, X. (2013). Chronic disease and the link to physical activity. *Journal of Sport and Health Science, 2*(1), 3-11. https://doi.org/10.1016/j.jshs.2012.07.009

Hamilton, M. T., Healy, G. N., Dunstan, D. W., Zderic, T. W., & Owen, N. (2008). Too little exercise and too much sitting: Inactivity physiology and the need for new recommendations on sedentary behavior. *Current Cardiovascular Risk Reports,* 2(4), 292-298. https://doi.org/10.1007/s12170-008-0054-8

Interprofessional Education Collaborative Expert Panel. (2011). Core competencies for interprofessional collaborative practice: Report of an expert panel. Washington, D.C.: Interprofessional Education Collaborative.

Jacobs, P.L. (2018). Rationale and considerations for training special populations in P.L. Jacobs (Ed) *NSCA's essentials of training special populations*. Champaign, IL: Human Kinetics.

Lobelo, F., Stoutenberg, M., & Hutber, A. (2014). The exercise is medicine global health initiative: A 2014 update. *British Journal of Sports Medicine, 48*(22), 1627-1633. https://doi.org/10.1136/bjsports-2013-093080

Mikeska, J. D. (2015). A SWOT analysis of the scope of practice for personal trainers. *Personal Trainer Quarterly, 2*(1), 22-25. Retrieved from http://www.nsca.com/education/articles/ptq/a-swot-analysis-of-the-scope-of-practice-for-personal-trainers/

Muth, N. D. (2007). Building the bridge: A career in medical fitness. *IDEA Fitness Journal, 4*(11), 56-63. Retrieved from http://www.ideafit.com/fitness-library/building-bridge-careermedical-fitness

Pedersen, B. K., & Saltin, B. (2015). Exercise as medicine—evidence for prescribing exercise as therapy in 26 different chronic diseases. *The Authors. Scandinavian Journal of Medicine & Science in Sports, 25* Suppl 3, 1-72. https://doi.org/10.1111/sms.12581

Spivey, K. (2015). Role and scope of practice for the certified medical exercise specialist in J.S. Skinner, C.X. Bryant, S. Merrill, & D.J. Green (Eds), *American Council on Exercise medical exercise specialist manual.* San Diego, CA: American Council on Exercise.

The National Institute of Diabetes and Digestive and Kidney Diseases. (2017). Overweight and obesity statistics. Retrieved from https://www.niddk.nih.gov/health-information/health-statistics/overweight-obesity

Tinetti, M. E., Fried, T. R., & Boyd, C. M. (2012). Designing health care for the most common chronic condition—multimorbidity. *JAMA, 307*(32), 2493-2494. https://doi.org/10.1001/jama.2012.5265

Twenge, J. M., & Campbell, W. K. (2018). Associations between screen time and lower psychological well-being among children and adolescents: Evidence from a population-based study. *Preventive Medicine Reports, 12*, 271-283. https://doi.org/10.1016/j.pmedr.2018.10.003

van Dongen, J. J., Lenzen, S. A., van Bokhoven, M. A., Daniels, R., van der Weijden, T., & Beurskens, A. (2016). Interprofessional collaboration regarding patients' care plans in primary care: A focus group study into influential factors. *BMC Family Practice, 17*, 58. https://doi.org/10.1186/s12875-016-0456-5

Waters, H., & Graf, M. (2018). The cost of chronic diseases in the U.S.: Executive summary. Washington, DC: Milken Institute.

Williamson, W. A. (2010). Medical exercise positioning: A business tool kit. *ACSM's Health & Fitness Journal, 14*(1), 30-33. https://doi.org/10.1249/FIT.0b013e3181c654d4

World Health Organization. (2010). *Framework for action on interprofessional education & collaborative practice*. Geneva: World Health Organization.

Weinstein, S. I., Yelin, E. H., & Watkins-Castillo, S. I. (2015). Chronic joint pain. United States. Bone and Joint Initiative. Retrieved from http://www.boneandjointburden.org/2014-report/ib2/chronic-joint-pain

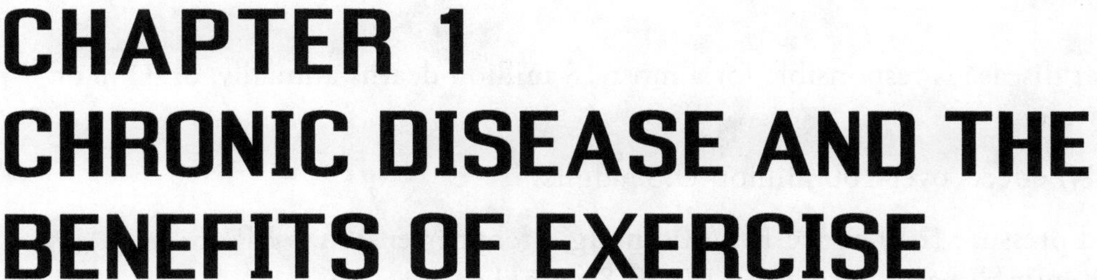

CHAPTER 1
CHRONIC DISEASE AND THE BENEFITS OF EXERCISE

By the end of this chapter you will understand:

- Exercise and chronic disease
- Exercise in the health care continuum
- Common terms
- FITT
- The three stages of prevention

Chronic Disease Statistics

Chronic disease is defined as a disease that progresses slowly, lasts for a year or longer, requires ongoing medical care, and interferes with activities of daily living (ADLs), versus *acute* disease that develops and dissipates quickly (Boothe, Roberts, & Laye, 2012). Most chronic diseases are caused by a few risk behaviors such as smoking, poor nutrition, excessive alcohol consumption, and a lack of physical activity. Whereas historically infection was the leading cause of death in the United States, today most people in the United States will die from chronic disease. The following statistics are alarming:

- Chronic diseases account for almost 70% of all deaths in the U.S., and interfere with activities of daily living for about 10% of the U.S. population.
- At least 50%, and maybe as many as 60% of the adult U.S. population has at least one chronic disease.

- 25-40% of the adult U.S. population have two or more chronic diseases.
- Almost 10% of the U.S. population has diabetes.
- Almost 40% of U.S. adults are considered obese.
- The most prevalent chronic disease is cardiovascular disease:
    - o Cardiovascular disease is a broad term for any disease of the heart, blood vessels, or circulation.
    - o Cardiovascular disease is responsible for almost 18 million deaths annually, or 31% of deaths worldwide.
- Hypertension (HTN) effects over 100 million U.S. adults.
    - o HTN is blood pressure (BP) above 140/90mmHg, prehypertension is BP of 120-130/80-89mmHg, and normal BP is 120/80mmHg.
- Type 2 diabetes effects over 30 million adults in the U.S. and is expected to increase to 336 million adults worldwide by 2030.
- In the U.S. 30 million adults suffer from osteoarthritis:
    - o It is thought that everyone over the age of 60 has at least one joint effected by osteoarthritis.
    - o Rheumatoid arthritis effects just 1% of the adult population.
- *Cancer* is the name given to a group of diseases characterized by uncontrolled cell growth that invade and degrade surrounding fresh tissue.
    - o Almost 2 million people in the U.S. are diagnosed with cancer annually, and almost 600,000 will die from it, making it the second leading cause of death.
- The prevalence of asthma has increased over the past few decades to just under 10% of the adult and child U.S. population.
- Physical activity can positively affect over 30 chronic conditions, making it the best deterrent of chronic disease in primary and secondary prevention.
- Only 15-20% of U.S. adults meet the minimum guidelines for physical activity.
- One-third of the world's population does not perform the recommended amount of daily activity, making a sedentary lifestyle one of the biggest public health threats of modern times (American Diabetes Association, 2019; American Heart Association, 2018; Boothe et al., 2012; Centers for Disease Control and Prevention (CDC), 2018; CDC, 2019a; CDC, 2019b; CDC, 2019c; CDC, 2019d; Durstine, Gordon, Wang, & Luo, 2013; Jacobs, 2018; Lobelo, Stoutenberg & Hutber, 2014; Pedersen & Saltin, 215; Philips & Kennedy, 2012; Spivey, 2015; World Health Organization, 2019).

Common Terms

Before we move on, there are a few terms that are often used interchangeably, and need to be defined (American College of Sports Medicine [ACSM], 2018; Booth et al., 2012; Fahey, Insel, & Roth, 2015).

- *Physical activity* is any bodily movement produced by voluntarily contracting skeletal muscle that results in energy expenditure above a basal level.
- *Exercise* is a repetitive and purposeful, planned, structured physical activity with the objective to improve or maintain one or more components of physical fitness, to include aerobic capacity, muscular strength, muscular endurance, flexibility, or agility.
- *Health* is the overall condition of the body or mind, and the presence or absence of illness or injury. Age, genetics, and family history can determine health, and therefore health may not always be controllable.
- *Wellness* encompasses a number of dimensions of well-being as a descriptor of optimal health. The dimensions are physical, emotional, financial, cultural, spiritual, intellectual, and interpersonal. Wellness is considered controllable based on the elimination of risk factors, diet, activity, and outlook or perception.
- *Physical inactivity* describes individuals who do not get the recommended amount of regular physical activity.
- *Clinical exercise*, *medical exercise*, and *medical fitness* are often used interchangeably, depending on the author of a text or study. We have tried to exclusively use the term *clinical exercise*, but if citing another author's work, we use the term the original author used.

FITT

Current guidelines for physical activity are based on the FITT template (frequency, intensity, time, type). The ACSM (2018) suggests moderate intensity aerobic exercise should be performed at least 5 days per week, and vigorous intensity activity be performed 3 days per week, or a combination of both. Moderate intensity aerobic activity is considered a VO_2 reserve (VO_2R) of 40-59%, and vigorous is considered a VO_2R of 60-84%. Bouts of moderate intensity aerobic exercise should last 30-60 minutes with a minimum of 150 minutes per week, and bouts of vigorous intensity aerobic exercise should last 20-60 minutes for at least 75 minutes per week. Aerobic exercise is considered rhythmic exercise using large muscle groups (Garber et al., 2011).

Resistance training should be performed 2-3 non-consecutive days per week. Starting intensity should be 40-50% of the maximum weight an individual can lift for one repetition (1RM), and progress to 60-80% for intermediate exercisers, and >80% for experienced exercisers. Although there are no time guidelines for resistance training, chosen exercises should target each major muscle group. Two-four sets are recommended, with 8-12 repetitions in each set for most adults, 10-15 repetitions for deconditioned adults, and 15-20 repetitions to improve muscular endurance (Garber et al., 2013).

Neuromuscular training should be performed 2-3 days per week with each bout lasting 20-30 minutes. Intensity guidelines for neuromuscular training have not been established, but exercises that challenge motor skills and proprioception should be performed.

Flexibility exercises should be done 2-3 days per week, but performing them more often increases the benefits. Each stretch should be taken to a point of tightness or slight discomfort, with static stretches held for 20-30 seconds, keeping in mind holding each stretch for longer offers increased benefits. Active, passive, dynamic, and proprioceptive neuromuscular facilitation (PNF) stretching are considered effective modalities. Table 1.1 details FITT protocols for apparently healthy adults.

Table 1.1

FITT guidelines

Mode	Frequency	Intensity	Time	Type
Cardiorespiratory Exercise/Aerobic	≥ 5 days/week of moderate intensity or ≥ 3 days/week of vigorous intensity	Moderate or vigorous	30-60 min/day of moderate (150 min/week) 20-60 min/day of vigorous (75 min/week)	Continuous, rhythmic, includes all major muscle groups
Older or deconditioned individuals		Light to moderate	bouts of <10 min can be beneficial	
Resistance Exercise	Each major muscle group 2-3 days/week	60%–70% of the 1RM (moderate to hard intensity) for novice to intermediate exercisers ≥80% of the 1RM (hard to very hard intensity) for experienced strength trainers <50% of the 1RM for muscular endurance	8–12 reps to improve strength 15–20 reps to improve muscular endurance 2-4 sets	Resistance exercises involving each major muscle group, targeting larger groups first
Older or deconditioned individuals		Light intensity; 40-50% 1RM	10–15 reps for strength 15-20 reps for muscular endurance A single set can be effective	
Posture Restoration	1-2x/day	Small overload in controlled positions	Hold isometric contractions for 5-10 seconds Dynamic contractions: 1-2 sets, 12-20 reps	30-45 minutes 1-3 months

Flexibility	≥ 2-3 days/week	Stretch to the point of feeling tightness or slight discomfort	Static stretching hold for 10-30 sec. or up to 60 sec. for older individuals For PNF stretching, a 3- to 6-sec contraction at 20%–75% maximum voluntary contraction followed by a 10-30 sec. assisted stretch	Static flexibility, Dynamic flexibility PNF
Older or deconditioned individuals			Static stretching hold for up to 60 sec.	
Posture Restoration	10 min bouts 1-2x/day	Static-to the point of tension Dynamic-controlled to the point of resistance	Static—2-4 reps; 30-60 seconds Dynamic—1-2 sets, 5-10 reps	30-45 min 1-3 months
Neuromuscular exercise training The effectiveness of neuromuscular exercise training in younger and middle-aged persons has not been Established	≥2-3 days/week	N/A	≥20-30 min/bout	Exercise that challenges motor skills, coordination, and proprioception such as Yoga or Tai Chi

Garber et al, 2011

Booth et al. (2012) suggest physical inactivity is activity at a level less than what is required for optimal health and is considered a cause of chronic disease and premature death. The deleterious effects of inactivity are progressive and compounding, resulting in a worse state of disease and/or dysfunction. Cardiovascular disease, muscular atrophy, hypertension, lipid disorders, diabetes, and osteoporosis will all deteriorate with prolonged periods of inactivity (Jacobs, 2018). In other words: use it or lose it.

Clinical Exercise in the Healthcare Continuum

The current model of healthcare in the U.S. is based on treatment rather than prevention (Ali & Katz, 2015). Treatment is given for a disease or injury that has been diagnosed; prevention is taking measures to avoid or improve a probable or possible disease or injury (Booth et al., 2012). Prevention is categorized as primary, secondary, or tertiary. The goal of primary prevention is to keep a condition from developing and includes immunizations, targeted types of exercise, wellness programs, and education. Secondary prevention interrupts the progression of disease to slow down or reverse the progression. Examples are treatment for hypertension, asthma, and some cancer treatments. The goal of tertiary prevention is to manage and treat symptomatic disease to reduce the severity, restore function, and reduce disease related complications, and includes treatment for late stage cancer, coronary heart disease, and rehabilitation (Boothe et al., 2012; Katz & Ali, 2009; Spivey, 2015). The best deterrent of chronic disease is physical activity for primary and secondary prevention; therefore, the main goal of clinical exercise in the health-care continuum is to prevent the onset of chronic disease (Durstine, et al., 2013).

The role of a clinical exercise specialist (CXS) is to work with a client's team of other healthcare providers. Building a medical network indicates a fitness professional's main goal is the wellbeing of a client. The team of providers may include a nutritionist or RD, a rehabilitation specialist or physical therapist, or an alternative healthcare provider such as a massage therapist or chiropractor. A client's referring physician may be a cardiologist, oncologist, or orthopedist; regardless, the physician is the center of the client's healthcare team and should be provided regular updates as to the client's progress (Mikeska, 2015; Spivey, 2015).

Discussion and application

1. Define chronic illness and provide an overview of how your fitness practice will benefit clients with one or more chronic illness. If possible, provide an example of how you have already done this.

2. Explain the three levels of prevention and provide examples of each one. How would you explain this to a client?

References

Ali, A., & Katz, D. L. (2015). Disease prevention and health promotion: How integrative medicine fits. *American Journal of Preventive Medicine, 49(*5 0 3), S230–S240. https://doi.org/10.1016/j.amepre.2015.07.019

American College of Sports Medicine. (2018). *ACSM's resources for the exercise physiologist: A practical guide for the health fitness professional* (P. Magyari, R. Lite, M. W. Kilpatrick, & J. E. Schoffstall Eds. 2 ed.). Philadelphia, PA: Wolters Kluwer.

American Diabetes Association. (2019). Statistics about diabetes. Retrieved from http://www.diabetes.org/diabetes-basics/statistics/.

American Heart Association. (2018). More than 100 million Americans have high blood pressure, AHA says. Retrieved from https://www.heart.org/en/news/2018/05/01/more-than-100-million-americans-have-high-blood-pressure-aha-says

Booth, F. W., Roberts, C. K., & Laye, M. J. (2012). Lack of exercise is a major cause of chronic diseases. *Comprehensive Physiology, 2*(2), 1143-1211. https://doi.org/10.1002/cphy.c110025

Centers for Disease Control and Prevention. (2018). Adult obesity facts. Retrieved from https://www.cdc.gov/obesity/data/adult.html.

Centers for Disease Control and Prevention. (2019a). About chronic disease. Retrieved from https://www.cdc.gov/chronicdisease/about/index.htm

Centers for Disease Control and Prevention. (2019b). Data, statistics, and surveillance: Asthma surveillance data. Retrieved from https://www.cdc.gov/asthma/asthmadata.htm

Centers for Disease Control and Prevention. (2019c). Health and economic cost of chronic disease. Retrieved from https://www.cdc.gov/chronicdisease/about/costs/index.htm

Centers for Disease Control and Prevention. (2019d). Osteoarthritis. Retrieved from https://www.cdc.gov/arthritis/basics/osteoarthritis.htm

Durstine, J. L., Gordon, B., Wang, Z., & Luo, X. (2013). Chronic disease and the link to physical activity. *Journal of Sport and Health Science, 2*(1), 3-11. https://doi.org/10.1016/j.jshs.2012.07.009

Garber, C. E., Blissmer, B., Deschenes, M. R., Franklin, B. A., Lamonte, M. J., Lee, I. M.,…Swain, D. P. (2011). Quantity and quality of exercise for developing and maintaining cardiorespiratory, musculoskeletal, and neuromotor fitness in apparently healthy adults: Guidance for prescribing exercise. *Medicine and Science in Sports Exercise, 43*(7), 1334-1359. https://doi.org/10.1249/MSS.0b013e318213fefb

Jacobs, P.L. (2018). Rationale and considerations for training special populations in P.L. Jacobs (Ed) *NSCA's essentials of training special populations*. Champaign, IL: Human Kinetics.

Katz, D. L., & Ali, A. (2009). Preventive medicine, integrative medicine & the health of the public [PDF]. Commissioned for the Institute of Medicine Summit on Integrative Medicine and the Health of the Public, 1-45.

Lee, I. M., Shiroma, E. J., Lobelo, F., Puska, P., Blair, S. N., & Katzmarzyk, P. T. (2012). Effect of physical inactivity on major non-communicable diseases worldwide: An analysis of burden of disease and life expectancy. *The Lancet, 380*(9838), 219-229. https://doi.org/10.1016/s0140-6736(12)61031-9

Lobelo, F., Stoutenberg, M., & Hutber, A. (2014). The exercise is medicine global health initiative: A 2014 update. *British Journal of Sports Medicine, 48*(22), 1627-1633. https://doi.org/10.1136/bjsports-2013-093080

Mikeska, J. D. (2015). A SWOT analysis of the scope of practice for personal trainers. *Personal Trainer Quarterly, 2*(1), 22-25. Retrieved from http://www.nsca.com/education/articles/ptq/a-swot-analysis-of-the-scope-of-practice-for-personal-trainers/

Pedersen, B. K., & Saltin, B. (2015). Exercise as medicine—evidence for prescribing exercise as therapy in 26 different chronic diseases. *Scandinavian Journal of Medicine & Science in Sports, 25* (Suppl 3), 1-72. https://doi.org/10.1111/sms.12581

Phillips, E. M., & Kennedy, M. A. (2012). The exercise prescription: A tool to improve physical activity. *Physical Medicine and Rehabilitation, 4*(11), 818-825. https://doi.org/10.1016/j.pmrj.2012.09.582

Spivey, K. (2015). Role and scope of practice for the certified medical exercise specialist in J.S. Skinner, C.X. Bryant, S. Merrill, & D.J. Green (Eds), *American Council on Exercise medical exercise specialist manual.* San Diego, CA: American Council on Exercise.

World Health Organization. (2019). Cardiovascular disease. Retrieved from https://www.who.int/cardiovascular_diseases/en/

CHAPTER 2
SCOPE OF PRACTICE AND HEALTH RISK

By the end of this chapter you will understand:

- The scope of practice for a clinical exercise specialist
- The on-boarding process (pre-participation screening) for a new client
- The importance of a paper trail to include a PAR-Q, a health history, the informed consent, and physician clearance

Scope of Practice

A basic personal training certification allows a personal trainer to work with apparently healthy clients. If a certified personal trainer (CPT) works with a client who has a chronic disease, a trainer may be outside the scope of practice. Because of the high prevalence of overweight and obesity, and the incidence of adults suffering from one or more chronic disease, chances are many CPTs work outside of their scope of practice (Mikeska, 2017).

When a trainer accepts a client, the client assumes a safe workout will be provided and there will be no undue stress or a risk of injury (Abbott, 2012). By offering advice that falls outside the scope of practice, a trainer and a facility may be open to a lawsuit. *Scope of practice* refers to professional boundaries based on knowledge skill, and abilities (KSAs), and is usually determined by education, experience, and demonstrated competency, such as a program of study, or an exam to measure proficiency (Abbott, 2012; Mikeska, 2015). A clinical exercise specialist (CXS) has the KSAs to conduct pre-participation interviews, perform fitness assessments, and design and implement health and fitness programs for disease management, that avoid future injury, and to improve activities of daily living (Galati, 2015). Although the scope of practice of many allied healthcare fields overlap, and many personal trainers admit to working with clients outside of their scope of practice (Abbott, 2012; Mikeska, 2017), a CXS is not a licensed healthcare provider and may not diagnose an unknown condition, design meal plans, suggest supplements, physically touch a client, or provide behavioral counseling (Mikeska, 2015; Spivey, 2015). Some KSAs associated with a CXS are:

- Knowledge of basic chronic disease pathophysiology.
- The use and side effects of common medications taken by someone suffering from a chronic disease.
- The knowledge to perform and analyze basic assessments related to movement and anthropometry.
- The knowledge to design a safe and effective workout based on information received via assessment results, and the clinical recommendations from other healthcare providers.
- FITT protocols, exercise progressions, and regressions.
- The implications of exercise and activity for individuals with chronic disease.
- Contraindications of chronic disease, and signs and symptoms of distress related to chronic disease.
- Knowledge of signs and symptoms that require expertise outside of the scope of practice for a CXS.
- The ability to recognize a medical emergency.
- The ability to administer adult CPR and AED.

Pre-participation Screening

A pre-participation screening is one of the best methods to ensure adherence to scope of practice protocols. The purpose of a pre-participation screening is to determine if a client has any contraindications prior to starting an exercise program. Even though all activity and exercise have inherent risks, the risks can be minimized by identifying and defining problems that may not be present during daily activity but may present during moderate or vigorous exercise. According to the American College of Sports Medicine (American College of Sports Medicine [ASCM], 2018), pre-participation screening can identify participants with medical contraindications, indicate participants who need to obtain a medical clearance, and identify participants who fall outside the scope of practice of a CXS (ACSM, 2018; Mikeska, 2017). Questionnaires should include a health history, a pre-activity risk stratification questionnaire, and if appropriate, a medical clearance (ACSM, 2018; Magal & Riebe, 2016; Tsai, 2015).

Par-Q vs. Physical Activity Risk Stratification

A pre-activity readiness questionnaire (PAR-Q) is a short medical questionnaire that provides minimal health information and can be used for clients who will perform low-moderate exercise. The original PAR-Q was seven questions; however, many in the medical community were concerned about its validity due to little evidence-based research, and some thought the simplistic questions led to false positives, and consequently, too many medical referrals (Bredin, Gledhill, Jamnik, & Warburton, 2013). The mentioned concerns led to the creation of the Physical Activity Readiness Questionnaire for Everyone, or PAR-Q+, which is a 4-page questionnaire, and starts with seven questions similar to original PAR-Q, but based on the answers, has follow-up questions to determine the need for medical clearance. A comparison of the initial questions is in Table 2.1

Table 2.1

PAR-Q vs. PAQ-Q+

PAR-Q	PAR-Q+
Has your doctor ever said that you have a heart condition and that you should only perform physical activity recommended by a doctor?	Has your doctor ever said that you have a heart condition or high blood pressure
Do you feel pain in your chest when you perform physical activity?	Do you feel pain in your chest at rest, during your daily activities of living, OR when you do physical activity?
In the past month, have you had chest pain when you were not performing any physical activity?	Do you lose balance because of dizziness, OR have you lost consciousness in the past twelve months. Please answer NO if your dizziness was associated with over-breathing (including vigorous activity)?
Do you lose your balance because of dizziness or do you ever lose consciousness?	Have you ever been diagnosed with another chronic medical condition (other than heart disease or high blood pressure)?
Do you have a bone or joint problem that could be made worse by a change in your physical activity?	Are you currently taking prescribed medications for a chronic medical condition?
Is your doctor currently prescribing any medication for your blood pressure or for a heart condition?	Do you have a bone or joint problem that could be made worse by becoming more physically active? Please answer NO if you had a joint problem in the past, but it does not limit your current ability to be physically active. For example, knee, ankle, shoulder, or other.
Do you know of any other reason you should not engage in physical activity?	Has your doctor ever said that you should only do medically supervised physical activity?

As you can see by the initial questions, the PAR-Q and PAR-Q+ are almost identical. Keep in mind, the one drawback to an overly conservative pre-participation screening is the negative effect of keeping asymptomatic individuals from participating in a beneficial exercise program, with the implication that a sedentary lifestyle is less of a risk than being active (Magal & Riebe, 2016; Thompson, Arena, Riebe, & Pescatello, 2013). Additionally, while the initial questions of the PAR-Q and PAR-Q+ are relevant to exercise capacity, they are not necessarily relevant to the risk of sudden death. Accordingly, ACSM has new pre-participation health screening recommendations (Magal & Riebe, 2016). Because exercise is safe for most people, and the absolute risk of a cardiovascular (CV) event is extremely low, as demonstrated by the list below (Magal & Riebe, 2016), it is thought previous guidelines were too conservative, with up to 95% of clients over age 40 advised to seek medical clearance.

- A single sudden cardiac death (SCD) occurs every 1.5 million episodes of vigorous physical exertion.

- A single SCD occurs every 36.5 million hours of moderate-to-vigorous exertion in women.
- Approximately 1 death occurs per 396,000 hours of jogging.
- Approximately 1 death occurs per 2,897,057 person-hours of exercise.
- Approximately 1 acute myocardial infarction (AMI) incident occurs per 184,000 runners.
- Approximately 1 SCD incident occurs per 256,000 runners.
- Approximately .20 AMI and 0.14 SCD per 100,000 estimated runner-hours.

The objective of the new guidelines is similar to the old (Magal & Riebe, 2016):

1. To identify individuals who should receive medical clearance before starting a new program or increasing the frequency, intensity, and/or volume of an existing exercise program.
2. To identify individuals who present with CV, metabolic, and/or renal diseases and will benefit from participating in a medically-supervised exercise program.
3. To identify individuals with CV, metabolic, and/or renal diseases who must wait until their medical condition(s) have improved to proceed with an exercise program.

However, individuals with pulmonary disease, joint or bone disease, or other non-life-threatening chronic conditions no longer need medical clearance to begin a light to moderate exercise program. Additionally, a recommendation to obtain medical clearance leaves the decision to perform a medically-supervised exercise test to a qualified physician, and not a CXS.

If your place of business requires the PAR-Q, PAR-Q+, or the electronic Physical Activity Readiness Medical Examination ePARmed-X+, you should comply with institutional protocols.

The sample Physical Activity Risk Stratification form (Appendix A) can be used as a guideline, or visit http://links.lww.com/FIT/A31 to download the pre-participation health screening form from ACSM. Other cardiovascular disease (CVD) risk factors that require close observation but may not prevent an individual from participating in an exercise program are listed in Table 2.2.

Table 2.2

CVD risk factors

Positive Risk Factor	Criteria
Age	Males 45 or older; Females 55 or older
Family History	Heart attack, coronary revascularization, or sudden death First degree relative: Male prior to 55 or female prior to 65 years of age
Cigarette Smoking	Within last 6 months, or subjected to secondhand smoke
Sedentary Lifestyle	NOT participating in 30 minutes of moderate-intensity activity 3 days/week for the last 3 months
Obesity	BMI 30 or higher. Waist circumference greater than 40" for males or 35" for females. Waist more than half of height
Hypertension	BP greater than 139/89, or currently on antihypertension medication
Dyslipidemia (Cholesterol)	LDL greater than 129, HDL less than 40, total greater than 200, or currently on medication
Pre-Diabetes/Diabetes	Fasting glucose greater than 99
Negative Risk Factor	Criteria
High Serum HDL	HDL greater than 60

Other signs and/or symptoms that indicate an exercise session should stop, be recorded, and details given to the client's physician are:

- Difficulty breathing
- Edema
- Tachycardia
- Pain or cramping in the lower legs (claudication)
- Unusual fatigue
- Dizziness

Health History

A health history questionnaire is usually completed after a PAR-Q, any CVD risk stratification, or the Physical Activity Risk Stratification form and provides valuable, detailed information for a CXS to develop an appropriate exercise program for a client with chronic disease. The form should include:

- Demographic information
    - Age
    - Sex
    - Marital status
- Exercise history
- Any medications and supplements
- Past or current illness or injuries
- Last medical exam
- Surgical history
- Known allergies
- Family medical history (Graham & Whitehead, 2018; Tsia, 2015)

Additional information related to lifestyle, employment, stress level, and attitude toward exercise and activity may also be beneficial to develop and implement a successful workout plan.

Informed Consent

Starting with the Hippocratic Oath and continuing today, ethics in medicine is a fundamental expectation of most people. The four principles of healthcare ethics are non-maleficence (do no harm), beneficence (do good to/for others), autonomy (self-determination and freedom of choice), and justice (equitable and fair treatment). Informed consent is based on the ethical principles of autonomy and beneficence (Schenker & Meisel, 2011).

Autonomy states an individual has the right to make choices without unnecessary influence or interference, while beneficence requires a participant will not be subjected to physical or psychological harm. Additionally, privacy and confidentiality are included under the principles of autonomy and beneficence (U.S. Department of Health & Human Services, n.d). Privacy specifies a participant will be free from unwarranted intrusion and allows participants to determine the extent of access others may have over them (autonomy). Confidentiality concerns with data, and how private data are controlled so potentially damaging information is not made public (beneficence).

An informed consent form should be completed by a client prior to any testing, program design, or the initiation of an exercise program. The form should contain information regarding the purpose and explanation of any assessments, any risks associated with participation, the expected benefits from participation, confidentiality controls and how information will be used and/or shared, and an acknowledgement that questions have been answered and a client fully understands the document. By signing an informed consent form, a client acknowledges the risks associated with the discussed activity and exercise plan, and is participating voluntarily (Graham & Whitehead, 2018).

Although having every client complete an informed consent is highly recommended, there is not an example of an informed consent or waiver included due to the variabilities across state and local laws. It is the responsibility of a CXS to seek legal advice from a qualified attorney.

A medical clearance form is not part of the pre-participation screening process, however, regardless of the necessity, it is recommended at some point, every client obtains medical clearance from a physician to evaluate any known medical conditions. For known CVD risk factors, follow the guidelines in the Physical Activity Risk Stratification form. The pre-participation screening and the medical clearance can provide information to effectively design a workout plan for clients with chronic disease, and to clarify goals, benefits, and risks. Additionally, the information can also prove invaluable for preparation if a medical emergency occurs. A sample medical clearance form can be found in Appendix B.

Discussion and application

1. What is the purpose of performing a pre-participation health screening (risk assessment), and what is involved?
2. How would you handle a client who ____________, and on what do you base your answer?
   a. Asks for nutrition advice
   b. Wants you to push on an overactive trigger spot
   c. Asks about knee or shoulder pain they may be experiencing

References

Abbott, A. A. (2012). The legal aspects: Scope of practice. *ACSM's Health and Fitness Journal, 16*(1), 31-34. https://doi.org/10.1249/FIT.0b013e31823d0452

American College of Sports Medicine. (2018). *ACSM's resources for the exercise physiologist: A practical guide for the health fitness professional* (P. Magyari, R. Lite, M. W. Kilpatrick, & J. E. Schoffstall Eds. 2 ed.). Philadelphia, PA: Wolters Kluwer.

Bredin, S. S. D., Gledhill, N., Jamnik, V. K., & Warburton, D. E. R. (2013). PAR-Q+ and ePARmed-X+: New risk stratification and physical activity clearance strategy for physicians and patients alike. *Canadian Family Physician, 59*(3), 273-277. Retrieved from https://www.ncbi.nlm.nih.gov/pmc/articles/PMC3596208/

Galati, T. (2015). Applying the ACE Integrated Fitness Training model in the medical exercise setting in J.S. Skinner, C.X. Bryant, S. Merrill, & D.J. Green (Eds), *American Council on Exercise medical exercise specialist manual.* San Diego, CA: American Council on Exercise.

Graham, J. F. & Whitehead, M. T. (2018). Health appraisal and fitness assessments in P.L. Jacobs (Ed) *NSCA's essentials of training special populations.* Champaign, IL: Human Kinetics.

Magal, M., & Riebe, D. (2016). New preparticipation health screening: What exercise professionals need to know. *ACSM's Health & Fitness Journal, 20*(3), 22-27. https://doi.org/10.1249/FIT.0000000000000202

Mikeska, J. D. (2015). A SWOT analysis of the scope of practice for personal trainers. *Personal Trainer Quarterly, 2*(1), 22-25. Retrieved from http://www.nsca.com/education/articles/ptq/a-swot-analysis-of-the-scope-of-practice-for-personal-trainers/

Mikeska, J. D. (2017). Continuous quality improvement to ensure personal training scope of practice. *Personal Trainer Quarterly, 4*(3), 24-28. https://www.nsca.com/uploadedFiles/NSCA/Resources/PDF/Publications/PTQ/PTQ%204.3.pdf

Schenker, Y., & Meisel, A. (2011). Informed consent in clinical care: Practical considerations in the effort to achieve ethical goals. *Journal of American Medical Association, 305*(11), 1130-1131. https://doi.org/10.1001/jama.2011.333

Spivey, K. (2015). Role and scope of practice for the certified medical exercise specialist in J.S. Skinner, C.X. Bryant, S. Merrill, & D.J. Green (Eds), *American Council on Exercise medical exercise specialist manual.* San Diego, CA: American Council on Exercise.

Thompson, P. D., Arena, R., Riebe, D., & Pescatello, L. S. (2013). ACSM's new preparticipation health screening recommendations from ACSM's guidelines for exercise testing and prescription, ninth edition. *Current Sports Medicine Reports, 12*(4), 15-17. https://doi.org/10.1249/JSR.0b013e31829a68cf

Tsia, N. T. (2015). Working with clients with health challenges in J.S. Skinner, C.X. Bryant, S. Merrill, & D.J. Green (Eds), *American Council on Exercise medical exercise specialist manual.* San Diego, CA: American Council on Exercise.

U.S. Department of Health & Human Services. (n.d.). The Belmont report: Ethical principles and guidelines for the protection of human subjects of research. Retrieved from http://www.hhs.gov/ohrp/humansubjects/guidance/belmont.html

CHAPTER 3
RAPPORT AND PSYCHOLOGY

By the end of this chapter you will understand:

- Psychological factors associated with chronic disease
- Stress
- Self-efficacy
- Models of behavior change
- The significance of building rapport with clients
- Client education
- SMART goal setting
- Shaping

As chronic disease becomes more prevalent, patients dealing with the stigma of chronic disease are seeking normalization (Joachim & Acorn, 2000). These conflicting concepts, stigma and normalization, have created a unique space in healthcare offering a proactive approach to reframe the social perspective. Accordingly, integrating behavior care into other forms of less stigmatizing health services is gaining attention as patients with chronic diseases seek allied providers to assist with lifestyle and disease management behaviors, and self-management support (Fisher & Dickinson, 2014). By understanding a client's perspective, a CXS can provide the support and a positive environment for clients to overcome or manage a chronic disease.

Understanding Stress

Up to 75% of Americans experience some type of stress in any given month (Clay, 2011). Stress can result in headaches, stomach problems, sleep disorders, anxiety, depression, weight disorders, irritability, cardiovascular disease, and much more. Dr. Hans Seyle (1950) described the stages of stress as a predictable, universal pattern, and termed the process the *General Adaption Syndrome*. Pleasant or unpleasant experiences can trigger stress. Pleasant stressors are termed *eustress*, and unpleasant stress is termed *distress*; the physical response to eustress and distress is the same.

- The first stage is alarm. The alarm stage is in response to the fight-or-flight reaction. Individuals in the alarm stage can experience physical and mental symptoms such as indigestion, headaches, depression, anxiety, weight gain, and sleep disorders.
- The second stage is resistance. During the resistance stage, the body learns to deal with stress, and can adapt to new levels of stress as it builds resistance.
- The final stage is exhaustion. As stress persists, life threatening exhaustion develops, that negatively effects physical and mental well-being.

Long term personality changes such as decreased extroversion, openness to experience, and conscientiousness have been associated with chronic disease (Jokela, Hakulinen, Singh-Manoux, & Kivimaki, 2014). Accordingly, as chronic disease persists, many iindividuals affected are stigmatized as they perceive themselves as damaged and discriminated against (Joachim & Acorn, 2000). However, individuals who find ways to adapt, and in many cases overcome chronic disease, begin the process of normalization as they resume previous responsibilities and duties. Normalization is the act of creating a positive attitude toward living with a chronic disease (Joachim & Acorn, 2000). As discussed, it is known exercise can help prevent (primary, secondary, and tertiary) of over 35 chronic conditions (Boothe, Roberts, & Laye, 2012).

Self-efficacy

Self-efficacy is the self-belief an individual is capable of executing behaviors necessary to achieve a goal (Carey & Forsyth, 2019). Clients who have strong self-efficacy will think of a new challenge as something to overcome, recover quickly from failure, and are committed. Clients with a low level of self-efficacy avoid new challenges and dwell on failures. Self-efficacy can be thought of as a cycle in behavior change, with past performance as the strongest predictor of success. Therefore, clients in the early stages of behavior change will naturally have a lower level of self-efficacy, and in later stages, self-efficacy will facilitate participation, and greater participation will, in turn, increase self-efficacy (Marcus, Selby, Niaura, & Rossi, 1992).

The pattern of attrition from exercise is similar to the relapse curve of heroin, alcohol, and tobacco use (Marcus et al., 1992). Accordingly, clients who feel they have not yet mastered an activity or exercise program, or are struggling with staying on schedule or experiencing disruptions, are at a greater risk for relapse than those in later stages of behavior change. Unfortunately, relapse will happen, and most likely with in the first 6 months. Understanding how behavior change is facilitated and taking measures to overcome barriers that may cause relapse will ensure continuation and continuity of a new client's exercise program.

Models of Behavior Change

When we talk with prospective clients it is important to understand their perspectives on their current behavioral patterns. Understanding will provide insights into how a CXS can prompt change in those patterns. Clients who are suffering from one or more chronic diseases may have a low level of self-esteem and self-confidence, they may suffer from depression and anxiety, as well as addiction or other negative coping mechanisms. The strategies and stages of the transtheoretical model of behavior change, the health belief model, and the self-determination theory may be useful to understand behavior change, and provide insights to overcome obstacles to client apprehension and to begin or continue an exercise program.

Transtheoretical Model

The transtheoretical model of behavior change provides strategies, based on stages of change, to determine readiness to make a change; accordingly, a program designed for an individual in one stage will not be effective for an individual in a different stage (Marcus et al., 1992; Prochaska & DiClemente, 2005; Rogers, 2015). The stages of the model are:

1. Precontemplation indicates an individual is unaware a problem can be solved. The goal is to help clients be mindful that the risk of doing nothing is greater than the risk of change by making the solution relevant to them. To accomplish this, there needs to be validation of a clients' circumstances, and clients need to be encouraged to seek information regarding their condition.

2. Contemplation occurs when a client is aware of a problem but does not know how to initiate change. In this stage, clients need to be informed of the options and provided some minimal direction. Clients need to understand the choice to change is theirs to make, be encouraged a positive outcome is possible and beneficial, and offered opportunities to begin the process.

3. Preparation is the stage when a client is ready to make a change and seeks opportunities to begin or increase activities related to change. Goals and priorities are established, and a structured program implemented. During preparation, clients need to receive positive feedback and reinforcement regarding the decision to change a behavior, and need to know if a problem arises, they are not alone.

4. Action indicates a client is acting autonomously, gaining a sense of self-liberation, and desiring opportunities to participate. The main goal in the action phase is to ensure changes become habit through emphasis on self-efficacy and long-term benefits. This is also the stage where a relapse is most likely to occur, therefore continual positive feedback and support are necessary.

5. Maintenance builds on the tools acquired during the first four stages. Plans are in place to overcome obstacles, and the client is capable of dealing with relapse. It is understood that maintenance requires fewer resources than building, and to avoid burn out, program variety should be encouraged.

Health Belief Model

The health belief model is predicated on variables of perception (Carpenter, 2010). The first is the belief people will begin healthy behaviors if they perceive that not doing so will have a negative effect; the stronger the belief, the greater the likelihood of initiating change. For behavior change to occur it is necessary to believe the change will bring about a drastic or strong positive result. Last, perceived barriers will prevent the adoption of the new behaviors. Barriers can include the seriousness of illness or injury, a lack of time, or a poor financial situation. Regardless, a client must perceive the benefits of an exercise program outweigh the barriers.

Self-determination Theory

The self-determination theory suggests there are three psychological needs, autonomy, competency, and relatedness, which facilitate behavior change (American College of Sports Medicine, 2018; Graham & Whitehead, 2018). Autonomy is the belief the decision to participate was a made freely by choice and without undue influence. Competence occurs when an individual successfully completes or masters an activity or exercise. Relatedness is defined as when an individual is connected to, or senses a belonging with, others. The extent to which these three psychological needs are met determines the level of motivation.

Motivation is described as intrinsic or extrinsic (Sebire, Standage, & Vansteenkiste, 2009). Extrinsic motivation is centered on achieving outward goals such as awards, respect of others, and money. Intrinsic goals are focused inward and may include moral achievements, values, and personal interests. For exercise, activity, and fitness, an extrinsically motivated client would be focused on losing weight or building muscle, while an intrinsically motivated client would be concerned with skill development, or health and wellness factors. Although the goals of each client need to be addressed, a client suffering from one or more chronic conditions is likely concerned with health and wellness, and therefore motivated by intrinsic factors. Additionally, the psychological needs described in the self-determination theory are considered intrinsic and need to be considered when developing an exercise program for a client with a chronic disease. Furthermore, while extrinsic feedback such as verbal cues are important during the initial stages of an exercise program, intrinsic feedback, based on experience, is provided by a client's internal voice, and is crucial for long-term commitment.

Rapport

A good client-CXS relationship begins with good communication. Unfortunately, communicating is not always easy, and can be more difficult for a client suffering from chronic disease as extroversion decreases, and irritability and interpersonal conflicts increase (Jokela et al., 2014). The first few minutes with a client are the most crucial time to build rapport, with the goal of fostering trust, and then compliance (Barkley, 2017). Rogers (2015) describes rapport as a mutual understanding and trust in a relationship, and is paramount to facilitate behavioral change. Initially, rapport can be established by spending a few, uninterrupted minutes focused completely on a client's needs. By understanding what is important to a client and discussing a program plan that addresses client concerns, the foundations of a positive environment of collaboration and teamwork can be built (Barkley, 2017).

Client concerns can include a lack of time, financial insecurity, or aches, pains, and failing physical ability. However, assuming the concerns of a client indicate a closed mind, and can lead to miscommunication and the failure to understand a client's needs or abilities, and ultimately failure due to false expectations. Allowing clients to explain, in their own words, and then reiterating their concerns back to them, displays empathy and provides a CXS an opportunity to address and clarify any foreseeable obstacles. It is best to do this in a quiet place with minimal distractions where focus can be placed on the client, and eye contact assured.

Educate Your Client

Recreation and fitness leaders lead by emphasizing skill instruction, educating for understanding, and facilitating change (Little & Watkins, 2004). Skill instruction involves leading by doing. An instructor shows how something can be done and encourages followers to imitate. Educating for understanding builds confidence by explaining the components of an activity, why it is performed, and how it benefits performers. The focus is on performers and their needs. Leading to facilitate change encompasses skill instruction and understanding, but the focus should be on personal change rather than a specific activity. The emphasis is on empowering clients to take the lessons and victories from an activity into other aspects of their lives. By using a combination of these leadership approaches, clients can get what they need, as well as what they want.

A method to ensure a client understands material is the teach-back method. With the teach-back method, sometimes called the show-me method, clients are asked to explain in their words what they need to know or do (Agency for Healthcare Research and Quality, 2015). The teach-back method has been demonstrated to improve understanding and adherence, reduce cancelled appointments, and improve satisfaction and outcomes.

Be SMART

Goal setting is a proven method to achieve behavior change (Bovend'Eerdt, Botell, & Wade, 2009); however, if expectations are too challenging or goals are too difficult, failure will most likely follow. The SMART method of goal setting allows for achieving realistic goals in a timely manner. The acronym SMART stands for:

- Specific goals—Setting a time or distance goal for cardiovascular exercise, eliminating unhealthy foods, or performing resistance weight training twice a week are examples of specific goals.
- Measurable goals—Setting a continuous 20-minute time goal for cardiovascular exercise, only eating pastry desserts on weekends, or bench pressing a certain weight are examples of measurable goals.
- Attainable goals—The goals should be within control. For example, running a marathon, or bench pressing 300 pounds may not be attainable goals for someone new to exercise.
- Relevant goals—Are the goals relevant to an individual? Does a client with arthritic knees need to run a marathon, or does a shoulder replacement client need to bench press twice their body weight?
- Time frame—A reasonable and realistic length of time should be allowed for goal achievement. For example, setting a time frame of 6 weeks to run a marathon is not a reasonable or realistic goal for a sedentary individual.

Shaping

Hope and fear are powerful motivators. Whereas fear is negative and leads to anxiety, hope is positive and leads to aspiration, and subsequently, long-term adherence. One way to convey hope is through shaping. Shaping is simply exercise progression via behavior change and affirmation (Rogers, 2015). Starting with achievable movements, based on assessments, a client slowly progresses to the ultimate goal. By beginning with an achievable exercise, a client is not overwhelmed or anxious, but gains hope and confidence. Shaping can then be used to slowly challenge a client to build new skills and develop new behaviors. Shaping is ideal for large goals that may take longer to achieve but can be divided into manageable segments. For example, running a marathon can be divided into the smaller goals of running a mile in 6 weeks, increasing to 3 miles in 6 months, and a marathon in 24-36 months.

A written contract is another powerful motivator to ensure long-term adherence. A contract is a voluntary and deliberate, binding agreement between two parties, or a self-agreement where expectations are written down, and mutually agreed upon. Using SMART goals to define the parameters of the contract may be a good place to start, but the agreement should be flexible enough to allow for adjustments as expectations and goals change. Regardless, to achieve goals, progress should be tracked, and the goals should be revised as needed.

Discussion and application

1. Why is rapport considered to be the foundation of any fitness program?
2. Taking into account the stigma and psychosocial effects of chronic disease, how would you encourage someone with a chronic condition to start an exercise program? If possible, use a real-life example of success and/or failure.

References

Agency for Healthcare Research and Quality. (2015). Health literacy universal precautions toolkit, 2nd Edition: Use the teach-back method: Tool #5. Retrieved from https://www.ahrq.gov/health-literacy/quality-resources/tools/literacy-toolkit/healthlittoolkit2-tool5.html

American College of Sports Medicine. (2018). *ACSM's resources for the exercise physiologist: A practical guide for the health fitness professional* (P. Magyari, R. Lite, M. W. Kilpatrick, & J. E. Schoffstall Eds. 2 ed.). Philadelphia, PA: Wolters Kluwer

Barkley, P. (2017). Building rapport with your patient: Positive case management outcomes. Caring. Retrieved from http://www.nahc.org/news/building-rapport-with-your-patient-positive-case-management-outcomes/

Booth, F. W., Roberts, C. K., & Laye, M. J. (2012). Lack of exercise is a major cause of chronic diseases. *Comprehensive Physiology, 2*(2), 1143-1211. https://doi.org/10.1002/cphy.c110025

Bovend'Eerdt, T. J., Botell, R. E., & Wade, D. T. (2009). Writing SMART rehabilitation goals and achieving goal attainment scaling: A practical guide. *Clinical Rehabilitation (23)*, 352-361. https://doi.org/10.1177/0269215508101741

Carey, M. P., & Forsyth, A. D. (2019). Teaching tip sheet: Self-efficacy. Retrieved from https://www.apa.org/pi/aids/resources/education/self-efficacy

Carpenter, C. J. (2010). A meta-analysis of the effectiveness of health belief model variables in predicting behavior. *Health Communication, 25*(8), 661-669. https://doi.org/10.1080/10410236.2010.521906

Clay, R. A. (2011). Stressed in America. *Monitor on Psychology, 42*(1), p. 60. Retrieved from https://www.apa.org/monitor/2011/01/stressed-america

Fisher, L., & Dickinson, W. P. (2014). Psychology and primary care: New collaborations for providing effective care for adults with chronic health conditions. *American Psychologist, 69*(4), 355-363. https://doi.org/10.1037/a0036101

Graham, J. F. & Whitehead, M. T. (2018). Health appraisal and fitness assessments in P.L. Jacobs (Ed) *NSCA's essentials of training special populations.* Champaign, IL: Human Kinetics.

Joachim, G., & Acorn, S. (2000). Living with chronic illness: The interface of stigma and normalization. *Canadian Journal of Nursing Research, 32*(3), 37-48. Retrieved from http://cjnr.archive.mcgill.ca/article/view/1589/1589

Jokela, M., Hakulinen, C., Singh-Manoux, A., & Kivimaki, M. (2014). Personality change associated with chronic diseases: Pooled analysis of four prospective cohort studies. *Psychological Medicine, 44*(12), 2629-2640. https://doi.org/10.1017/S0033291714000257

Little, D. E., & Watkins, M. N. (2004). Exploring variation in recreation activity leaders' experiences of leading. *Journal of Park & Recreation Administration, 22*(1). Retrieved from https://js.sagamorepub.com/jpra/article/view/1485

Marcus, B.H., Selby, V.C., Niaura, R.S., & Rossi, J.S. (1992). Self-efficacy and the stages of exercise behavior change. *Research Quarterly for Exercise and Sport, 63*(1), 60-66. https://doi.org/10.1080/02701367.1992.10607557

Prochaska, J. O., & DiClemente, C. C. (2005). The transtheoretical approach. In J. C. Norcross & M. R. Goldfried (Eds.), *Handbook of psychotherapy integration* (2nd ed., pp. 147-171). New York, NY: Oxford University Press Inc.

Rogers, T. (2015). Behavioral change in J.S. Skinner, C.X. Bryant, S. Merrill, & D.J. Green (Eds), *American Council on Exercise medical exercise specialist manual.* San Diego, CA: American Council on Exercise.

Sebire, S. J., Standage, M., & Vansteenkiste, M. (2009). Examining intrinsic versus extrinsic exercise goals: Cognitive, affective, and behavioral outcomes. *Journal of Sport and Exercise Psychology, 31*(2), 189-210. https://doi.org/10.1123/jsep.31.2.189

Seyle, H. (1950). Stress and the general adaptation syndrome. *British Medical Journal, 1*(4667), 1383-1392. https://doi.org/10.1136/bmj.1.4667.1383

CHAPTER 4 POSTURAL AND MOVEMENT ASSESSMENTS, & CORRECTIVE STRATEGIES

By the end of this chapter you will understand:

- The importance of stability and mobility
- Postural distortions
- Assessments
  - o Movement
  - o Overweight/Obesity
- Assessment/Solutions tables

As you read this chapter, keep in mind, the cause of some postural deviations and movement dysfunctions is correctable, such as dysfunction caused by repetitive motions or mobility/stability imbalances. Other dysfunctions such as structural anomalies or injuries caused by trauma or disease are not correctable.

Stability and Mobility

The first goal of any training program is to ensure activities of daily living can be performed. Five foundational movements, or a combination of the foundational movements, are primarily used to perform most activities: squatting, single leg movements such as lunges and walking, pushing, pulling, and rotating (Cook, Burton, & Hoogenboom, 2006; Galati, 2015). These movements require a level of stability and mobility. Overactive muscles will often result in limited mobility, while underactive muscles often result in poor stability. Kinetic stability is when posture or a joint remains unchanged or returns to proper alignment, even when resistance is applied (American College of Sports Medicine [ACSM], 2018; Comana & McGrath, 2015; Galati, 2015). Stability is achieved by a coordinated effort of muscle activation that creates stiffness around a joint. Mobility is articulation, and balance is the ability to maintain the center of gravity, statically or dynamically, over the base of support (Comana & McGrath, 2015; Galati, 2015). Remembering stability requires little range of motion compared to mobility, and starts with the ground, will help to understand which joints provide stability and which provide mobility. Muscular imbalance occurs when mobility joints are used for stability, and stability joints are used for mobility. Figure 4.1 details the primary function of each joint or skeletal segment, and Figure 4.2 displays how altered kinematics and dysfunction in one area leads to compensatory movements in another.

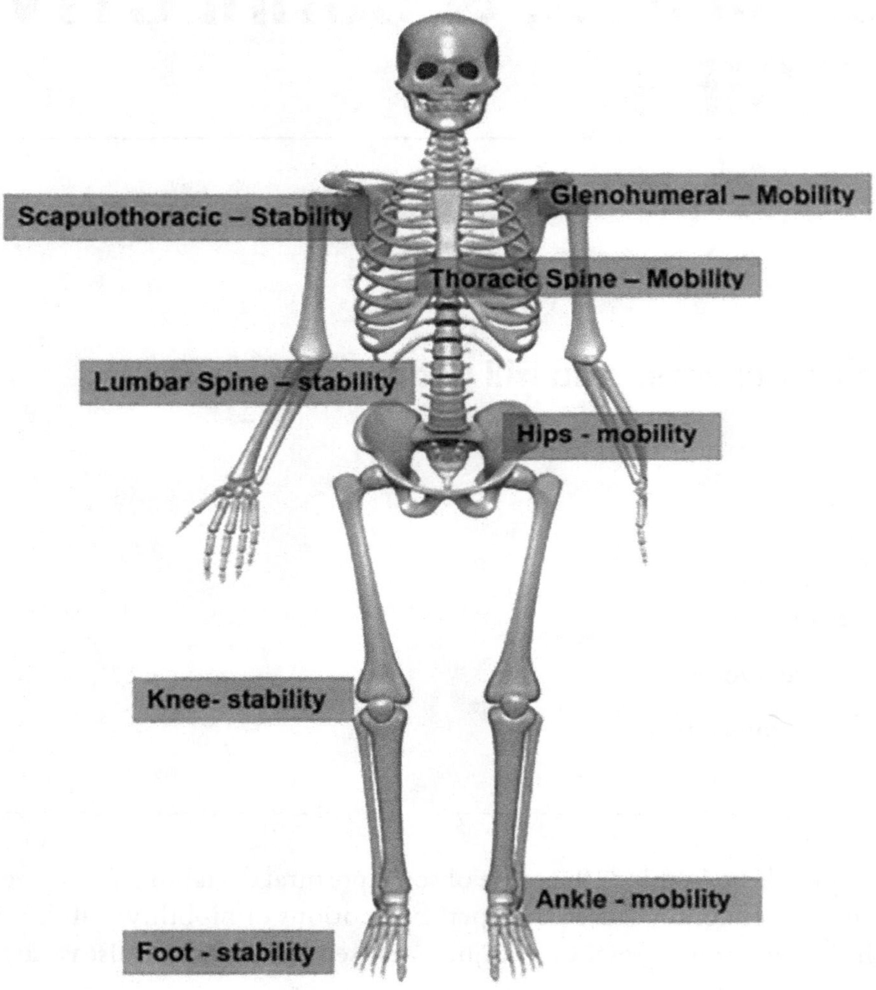

Figure 4.1 Stability and mobility. This figure details the primary function of each joint or skeletal segment.

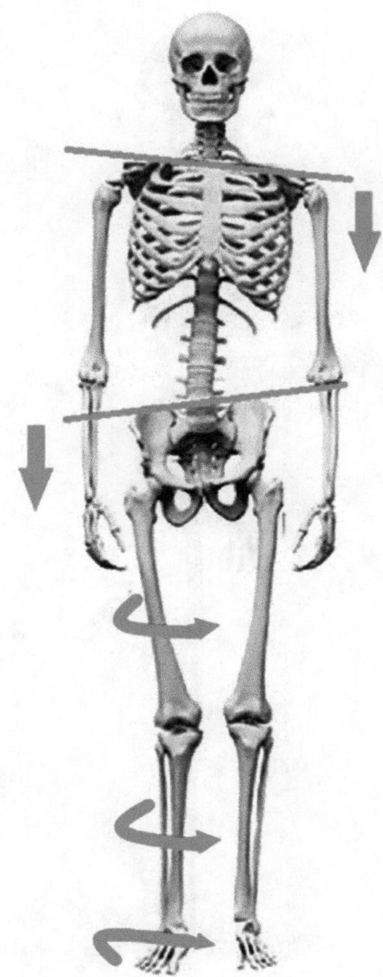

Figure 4.2 Altered kinematics. This figure displays how 4 degrees of dysfunction in one segment can affect the segments above and/or below.

Postural Distortions

Muscular imbalances result in impaired movement patterns and postural dysfunction. Proper posture requires the muscles and joints work minimally to maintain a state of musculoskeletal alignment and balance, and is indicated when a plumb line passes slightly in front of the ankle bone (lateral just in front of the center of the knee joint, through the greater trochanter, and then through the lumbar vertebrae and the center of the shoulder joint and ear as seen in Figure 4.3 (Norris, 2011).

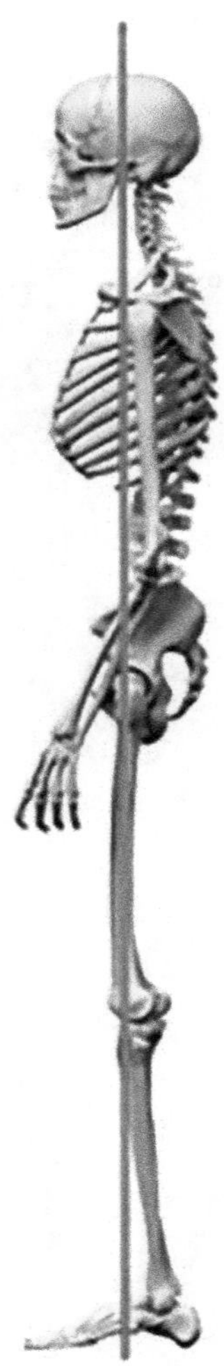

Figure 4.3 A plumbline can be used to determine proper static posture.

Static posture deviation manifests in four ways (not including scoliosis or lateral curvature of the spine) (Comana & McGrath, 2015: Norris, 2011).

1. Lordosis is indicated by an increased anterior curve.
2. Kyphosis is indicated by an increased posterior thoracic curve.
3. Flat back is indicated by a decreased lumbar curve.
4. Swayback is indicated by a decreased lumbar curve and an increased posterior thoracic curve.

In addition to the postural deviations already mentioned, Janda (1996) recognized patterns of overactive and underactive relationships that he termed proximal and distal crossed syndrome. This classification may be more useful to medical professionals, but the deviations are commonly encountered by fitness professionals and can often be corrected, so each has been renamed and explained by various fitness organizations. Proximal crossed syndrome has been relabeled *upper crossed* or *upper extremity syndrome*, and distal crossed syndrome has been relabeled *lower crossed syndrome* or *lumbo-pelvic-hip syndrome*. Upper crossed syndrome is characterized by a forward head and rounded shoulders. Lower crossed syndrome is characterized by increased lumbar lordosis and an anterior pelvic tilt. Another, although more recent postural deviation classification, is lower extremity, or pronation distortion syndrome. Pronation distortion syndrome is characterized by excessive foot pronation and knee flexion with internal rotation. Table 4.1 details common injuries associated with each distortion, as well as overactive and underactive muscles; Table 4.2 provides corrective strategies for postural distortions.

Table 4.1

Common postural distortions

Distortion	Common Injuries	Overactive	Under Active
Lower Extremity Pronation Distortion Syndrome	Plantar Fasciitis Posterior Tibialis Tendonitis (Shin Splints) Anterior Knee Pain Low Back Pain	Peroneal Gastrocnemius Soleus IT Band Hamstrings Adductors Iliopsoas	Posterior Tibialis Anterior Tibialis Vastus Medialis Gluteus Medius Gluteus Maximus
Upper Extremity Syndrome or Upper Crossed Syndrome	Rotator Cuff Impingement Shoulder Instability Biceps Tendonitis Thoracic Outlet Syndrome Headaches	Pectoralis Major Pectoralis Minor Levator Scap Teres Major Upper Trap Anterior Deltoid Subscapularis Lats Sternocleidomastoid Rectus Capitus Scalenes	Rhomboids Lower Trap Serratus Anterior Posterior Delt Teres Minor Infraspinatus Longus Coli/Capitus
Lumbo-Pelvic-Hip Syndrome or Lower Crossed Syndrome	Hamstring Strain • Anterior Knee Pain • Low Back Pain	Iliopsoas Rectus Femoris TFL Short Adductors Erector Spinae Gastrocnemius Soleus	Gluteus Maximus Hamstrings Gluteus Medius Transverse Abs Multifidus Internal Obliques Anterior and Posterior Tibialis

Table 4.2

Corrective strategies for postural distortions

Distortion	Compensation	Overactive	Under Active	Example Exercises
Lower Extremity-Pronation Distortion Syndrome Injuries: • Plantar Fasciitis • Posterior Tibialis Tendonitis (Shin Splints) • Anterior Knee Pain • Low Back Pain	• Excessive Foot Pronation • Knee Flexion/ Internal Rotation	Peroneal Gastrocnemius Soleus IT Band Hamstrings Adductors Iliopsoas	Posterior Tibialis Anterior Tibialis Vastus Medialis Gluteus Medius Gluteus Maximus	Strengthen: Dorsiflex w/band Mini squat-heel touch Ball Squat w/ Abduction S/L Bridge Kick Backs Stretch: Plantar Flex-Invert SMR Calf Calf Stretch SMR IT Band Sit and reach Lunge and Reach
Upper Extremity-Upper Cross Syndrome Common Injuries: • Rotator Cuff Impingement • Shoulder Instability • Biceps Tendonitis • Thoracic Outlet Syndrome • Headaches	• Rounded Shoulders • Forward Head	Pectoralis Major Pectoralis Minor Levator Scapula Teres Major Upper Trap Anterior Deltoid Subscapularis Latissimus Dorsi Sternocleidomastoid Rectus Capitus Scalenes	Rhomboids Lower Trap Serratus Anterior Posterior Deltoids Teres Minor Infraspinatus Longus Coli/ Capitus	Strengthen: 3-way rotator cuff Cobra Low Row Chin Tuck Stretch: Doorway Stretch Neck stretch Lat stretch O/B Kneeling Lat stretch
Lumbo-Pelvic-Hip-Lower Cross Syndrome Common Injuries: • Hamstring Strain • Anterior Knee Pain • Low Back Pain	Increased Lumbar Lordosis	Iliopsoas Rectus Femoris Tensor fasciae latae Short Adductors Erector Spinae Gastrocnemius Soleus	Gluteus Maximus Hamstrings Gluteus Medius Transverse Abs Multifidus Internal Obliques Anterior and Posterior Tibialis	Strengthen: S/L Bridge Ball Squat w/ Abduction Bracing Cobra O/B Dorsiflex w/band Crunch w/twist Stretch: SMR TFL SMR Calf TFL Stretch Calf Stretch Lunge Stretch w/ internal twist S/L Butterfly

Assessments

The overhead squat assessment

The overhead squat assessment (OHS) is a good starting point for screening a client's stability and mobility (Clifton, Grooms, & Onate, 2015; Hirth, 2007). It is not as comprehensive as the Functional Movement Screen (FMS) (Clifton, et al., 2015), but takes considerably less time to complete and provides enough information so any obvious movement dysfunction can be addressed. Additionally, the FMS was developed to determine the functional ability of athletes undergoing rehabilitation, and as such was not originally intended for clients suffering from one or more chronic disease, who may be unable to complete the seven movements of the FMS. Regardless, the OHS is only a basis for program design, and as you get to know your client, other concerns may arise that were unnoticed in the original assessment and may need to be addressed. To perform an OHS assessment, a client should stand with feet hip width apart, toes forward, and arms raised above the head. A CXS will view a number of squats from the front, back, and side. A client should perform the overhead squat as many times as needed so any movement imbalance can be recorded. Table 4.3 details what should be observed, and correction strategies (National Academy of Sports Medicine, n.d.)

Table 4.3

Overhead squat assessment chart

View	Checkpoint	Compensation	Possible injuries	Overactive	Under active
Anterior	Feet	Turns Out	Plantar Fasciitis Posterior Tibialis Tendonitis-shin splints Patellar Tendonitis-jumpers knee	Soleus Lat. Gastrocnemius Bicep Femoris Tensor Fascia Latae (TFL)	Med. Gastrocnemius Med. Hamstring Gluteus Med/Max Gracilis Sartorius Popliteus
	Knees	Move Inward	Anterior, medial, and lateral knee pain IT Band tendonitis	Adductor Complex Bicep Femoris (short head) TFL Lat. Gastrocnemius Vastus Lateralis	Med. Hamstring Med. Gastrocnemius Gluteus Med/Max Vastus Medialis (VMO)
		Move Outward		Piriformis Bicep Femoris TFL Gluteus Medius/ Minimus	Adductors Complex Med. Hamstring Gluteus Max

Lateral	LPHC	Excessive Forward Lean	Hamstring, quad, and groin strain Low back pain	Soleus Gastroc Hip Flexor Complex Abs	Anterior Tibialis Gluteus Max Erector Spinae
		Low Back Arches		Hip Flexor Complex Erector Spinae Latissimus Dorsi	Gluteus Maximus Hamstring Core Stabilizers (transverse abs, multifidus, transversospinalis, internal oblique, diaphragm, pelvic floor muscles)
		Low Back Rounds		Hamstrings Adductor Magnus Rectus Abdominis External Obliques	Gluteus Maximus Erector Spinae Lats/Psoas Intrinsic Core Stabilizers
	Upper Body	Arms Fall Forward	Headaches Biceps Tendonitis Shoulder Injuries	Latissimus Dorsi Pectoralis Major/ Minor Coracobrachialis Teres Major	Mid/Low Traps Rhomboids Posterior Deltoid Rotator Cuff
Posterior	Feet	Flatten	Plantar Fascitis Posterior Tibialis Tendonitis-Shin Splints Patellar Tendonitis-Jumpers Knee	Peroneal Complex (peroneus tertius, peroneus longus, peroneus brevis) Bicep Femoris TFL Lat. Gastrocnemius	Anterior/Posterior Tibialis Med. Gastrocnemius Gluteus Med Med. Hamstrings
		Heels Rise		Soleus	Anterior Tibialis
	LPHC	Asymmetrical Weight Shifting	Hamstring, Quad, Groin Strain Low Back Pain SI joint pain	Adductor Complex, TFL (on side of shift) Piriformis, Bicep Femoris (short head) Gluteus Medius (opposite of shift)	Gluteus Med-on side of shift Adductor Complex-on opposite side of shift

Overweight and obesity

In addition to movement and posture assessments, there are also a number of commonly used tools to assess obesity. Anthropometric measurements such as body fat percentage, body-mass index (BMI), and waist-to-hip ratios assess the size, shape, and composition of the human body. Body fat percentage can be measured in a number of ways inclding skin fold measurements, bioelectrical impedance, and hydrostatic weighing. Table 4.4 details body fat classifications (Kravitz, 2015).

Table 4.4

Body fat classifications

Classification	Males %	Females %
Essential fat	2-5	10-13
Athletes	6-13	14-20
Fitness	14-17	21-24
Average	18-24	25-31
Obese	>25	>32

The most prevalent anthropometric measurement for health risk is BMI that is used to categorize individuals from underweight to obese. BMI is a calculation of height and weight.

- [Body weight in pounds / (height in inches x height in inches)] x 703
- [Body weight in kg / (height in meters x height in meters)]

Underweight = <18.5
Normal Weight = 18.5-24.9
Overweight = 25.0-29.9
Obese = >30

The BMI scale has come under scrutiny as it does not differentiate between fat-free mass and fat mass. However, waist circumference can be used as an indicator for visceral fat, and a valid predictor of health risk (Janssen, Katzmarzyk, & Ross, 2004). Therefore, waist circumference measurements used as a separate indicator for health risk, and used in conjunction with BMI, can differentiate between healthy and unhealthy mass. For men, a waist of ≥ 40 inches (102cm), and for women a waist of ≥ 35 inches (89cm) are the thresholds for obesity related health risks.

Another measurement gaining popularity to assess cardiovascular risk is hip-to-waist ratio because it is more discriminate of lean vs. fat mass (Elsayed, et al., 2008). Measure at the smallest part of the waist, and the largest part of the hips and divide the waist the by hip measurement.

Table 4.5 details thresholds for waist-to-hip ratios.

Table 4.5

Hip to waist ratio

Gender	Excellent	Good	Average	Poor
Male	<0.85	0.85-0.89	0.90-0.95	>0.95
Female	<0.75	0.75-0.79	0.80-0.86	>0.86
Kravitz, 2015				

Discussion and application

1. Describe the mechanical dysfunction(s) associated with knee adduction and the movements needed to correct it. How can this be explained so a client will understand what is involved?
2. What imbalances exist for a client displaying kyphosis (upper-cross syndrome)? What exercises can be performed to alleviate the postural dysfunction? What cues can be suggested for a client to practice throughout the day?

References

American College of Sports Medicine. (2018). *ACSM's resources for the exercise physiologist: A practical guide for the health fitness professional* (P. Magyari, R. Lite, M. W. Kilpatrick, & J. E. Schoffstall Eds. 2 ed.). Philadelphia, PA: Wolters Kluwer.

Clifton, D. R., Grooms, D. R., & Onate, J. A. (2015). Overhead deep squat performance predicts functional movement screen score. *The International Journal of Sports Physical Therapy, 10*(5), 622-627. Retrieved from https://spts.org/member-benefits-detail/enjoy-member-benefits/journals/ijspt

Comana, F. & McGrath, C. (2015). Posture and movement in J.S. Skinner, C.X. Bryant, S. Merrill, & D.J. Green (Eds), *American Council on Exercise medical exercise specialist manual.* San Diego, CA: American Council on Exercise.

Cook, G., Burton, L., & Hoogenboom, B. (2006). Pre-participation screening: The use of fundamental movements as an assessment of function—part 1. *North American Journal of Sports Physical Therapy, 1*(2), 62-72. Retrieved from http://www.ncbi.nlm.nih.gov/pmc/articles/PMC2953313/

Elsayed, E. F., Tighiouart, H., Weiner, D. E., Griffith, J., Salem, D., Levey, A. S., & Sarnak, M. J. (2008). Waist-to-hip ratio and body mass index as risk factors for cardiovascular events in CKD. *American Journal of Kidney Disease, 52*(1), 49-57. https://doi.org/10.1053/j.ajkd.2008.04.002

Galati, T. (2015). Applying the ACE Integrated Fitness Training model in the medical exercise setting in J.S. Skinner, C.X. Bryant, S. Merrill, & D.J. Green (Eds), *American Council on Exercise medical exercise specialist manual.* San Diego, CA: American Council on Exercise.

Hirth, C. J. (2007). Clinical movement analysis to identify muscle imbalances and guide exercise. *Athletic Therapy Today, 12*(4), 10-14. Retrieved from http://www.scribd.com/doc/88697184/NASM-Clinical-Movement-Analysis-PDF-411K

Janda, V. (1996). Evaluation of muscular imbalance. In C. Leibenson (Ed.), *Rehabilitation of the spine: A practitioner's manual* (pp. 97-112). Baltimore, MD: Lippincott, Williams, and Wilkins.

Janssen, I., Katzmarzyk, P. T., & Ross, R. (2004). Waist circumference and not body mass index explains obesity-related health risk. *The American Journal of Clinical Nutrition, 79*(3), 379-384. https://doi.org/10.1093/ajcn/79.3.379

Kravitz, L. (2015). Overweight and obesity in J.S. Skinner, C.X. Bryant, S. Merrill, & D.J. Green (Eds), *American Council on Exercise medical exercise specialist manual.* San Diego, CA: American Council on Exercise.

National Academy of Sports Medicine. (n.d.) Overhead squat solutions table—CES. Retrieved from https://www.nasm.org/docs/default-source/PDF/overhead_squat_solutions_table-(ces-version)-(pdf-40k).pdf?sfvrsn=2

Norris, C. (2011). Posture: Part 1. *SportEX Dynamics(28),* 11. Retrieved from http://www.magcloud.com/browse/issue/192066

Science for Fun. (2019). Skeletal system [jpeg image]. Retrieved from http://science4fun.info/skeletal-system/

CHAPTER 5 CARDIORESPIRATORY ASSESSMENT

By the end of this chapter you will understand:

- Common definitions
- Maximal vs. submaximal assessment
- Termination of the assessment/contraindications
- Metrics
    - o Ventilatory threshold
    - o Rating of perceived exertion (RPE) and the ventilatory response to exercise
    - o Talk test
- YMCA step test

Although, as discussed in Chapter 1, the recommended amount of moderate intensity aerobic activity or exercise is 150 minutes per week (Garber et al., 2011), it is important to remember that if a client has been sedentary or is deconditioned, the main goal of a beginning aerobic program is to improve function by reversing physical deconditioning, improve physical function, improve activities of daily living, and increase health and well-being (Durstine et al, 2000). The prescribed exercise should induce the desired response without inducing any abnormal reactions. In the early stages of training, a deconditioned client may only be able to achieve a few minutes of exercise at a time, making any assessment difficult. The American Council on Exercise (Galati, 2015) suggests clients at this base-level of training do not need to perform a cardiorespiratory assessment until they are comfortable with the chosen assessment criteria and can sustain 20-minutes of cardiorespiratory activity. Intensity can be progressed when a client can maintain steady-state cardiorespiratory exercise for 20-30 minutes.

Definitions

Assessments are not meant to diagnose a medical condition, but rather to obtain a base level for program design, to track progress, and to give a CXS insights for exercise frequency, duration, and intensity. To avoid confusion of nomenclature, her are a few definitions:

- Heart rate reserve (HRR)—The difference between maximal heart rate and resting heart rate. It is based on the hearts ability to increase beats and output above a resting level, and indicates the reserve capacity of the heart.
- VO_2 max—Also referred to as maximal oxygen consumption, maximal oxygen uptake, or maximal aerobic capacity, is the maximum amount of oxygen used in 1 minute.
- VO_2 reserve (VO_2R)—The difference between VO_2 max and VO_2 at rest.
- Max heart rate—MHR (HRmax) is the highest heart rate that can be achieved.
- Target heart rate—Target heart rate or training heart rate, is the heart beats per minute used to determine training intensity.

Maximal vs. Submaximal

Aerobic assessments are used to determine VO_2max, which refers to the maximum amount of oxygen an individual uses during intense exercise and is considered the best measurement of cardiovascular capacity. If an assessment is performed, a maximal or submaximal test can be used. Maximal testing is considered the gold-standard to assess maximal aerobic capacity. A maximal test is usually performed on a bicycle or treadmill using a graded exercise protocol where the intensity increases as the test continues and stops when a client can no longer sustain the workload or continue the assessment. VO_2max is determined when oxygen consumption plateaus (Noonan & Dean, 2000).

Because maximal testing requires maximal exertion (Sartor et al., 2013), many clients who have chronic disease, an injury, or have been sedentary may not be able to perform a maximal aerobic assessment, and will need to perform a submaximal assessment. Submaximal assessments are often preferred over maximal tests because they can be measured in smaller increments, and the results are extrapolated based on predetermined norms. Submaximal assessments can also be performed on a variety of equipment allowing the test to be conducted in almost any setting as no special or expensive equipment is needed (Sartor et al., 2013). Examples of submaximal aerobic assessments are the modified Bruce treadmill test, the Rockport walk test, the timed up and go test, the YMCA cycle test, the Harvard step test, and the YMCA 3-minute step test. The guidelines for the YMCA 3-minute step test are located in Appendix C.

Termination of Assessment

Regardless of maximal or submaximal, some clients with physical limitations may never adequately perform an aerobic assessment. Risk factors that need to be considered with cardiorespiratory exercise include history of injury or disease, level of conditioning, and level of stability and mobility (American

College of Sports medicine [ACSM], 2018). Additionally, ACSM (2018) recommends stopping the assessment for any of the following reasons:

- Onset of angina or similar symptoms.
- Drop in SBP of ≥10mm Hg with an increase in work rate, or if SBP decreases below the value obtained in the same position prior to testing.
- SBP rises above 250mm Hg and/or DBP rises above 115mm Hg.
- Shortness of breath, wheezing, leg cramps, or claudication (lower leg cramps).
- Signs of light headedness, confusion, ataxia, pallor, nausea, or cold and clammy skin.
- Failure of HR to increase with increased exertion
- Noticeable change in heart rhythm, palpitations, or auscultation.
- Participant requests to stop.
- Physical or verbal manifestations of severe fatigue.
- Equipment failure.

Metrics

Ventilatory threshold

Many of the methods to determine the training heart rate based on HRmax can have a variance of up to +/- 14 beats/minute (Galati, 2015). When developing a cardiorespiratory training program for a client with chronic disease, a variance of 14 beats per minute can be detrimental to progression, or in the worst-case scenario, a client's health. Ventilation linearly increases with oxygen consumption and carbon dioxide production. Accordingly, there are two ventilatory threshold levels that can be determined via submaximal testing. The first ventilatory threshold (VT1, often referred to as lactate threshold or anaerobic threshold) is the point during exercise training at which ventilation is disproportionately high with respect to oxygen consumption as the body clears lactate in the blood. Breathing becomes labored and talking is difficult at VT1 and is usually reached at around 50–60% of peak VO_2 or 60–70% of peak heart rate (American Council on Exercise, n.d.; Mezzani et al., 2012). The second ventilatory threshold (VT2 or respiratory compensation threshold) occurs when blood lactate can no longer be effectively cleared and starts to accumulate. VT2 is recognized by heavy breathing and the inability to talk (many clients may never or should not attempt to achieve VT2), and is usually reached at 70–80%peak VO_2, and 80–90%peak heart rate (American Council on Exercise, n.d.; Mezzani et al., 2012).

Rating of perceived exertion and talk test

Because most gyms and fitness studios do not have expensive equipment for testing VO_2, there are a number of field tests that require no equipment, and can accurately determine VT1. Borg's Rating of Perceived Exertion (RPE) scale and the talk test (TT) have been determined to be valid indicators for VT1 (lactate, or anaerobic threshold). As discussed, VT1 occurs when breathing is slightly labored, and talking is possible but difficult (Woltmann et al., 2015). The TT is conducted by incrementally increasing the intensity of the exercise (treadmill, cycle, elliptical, etc.) until a performer can no longer recite a predetermined passage without compromising the integrity of the passage. The TT is easy to conduct and allows for individual programing. The RPE test is based on a scale of 6-20; 6 = no exertion and 20 = maximal exertion (ACSM, 2018). The RPE scale corresponds to metabolic markers and is easy to teach. An RPE of 11-13 corresponds to VT1 and is a recommended starting point for clients who are at a base level (Scherr et al., 2013). For some clients (and trainers) using an RPE scale of 0-10, 0 = no exertion, and 10 = maximal exertion, may be easier to understand. Using an RPE of 0-10, 3-4 corresponds to a base level just at or below VT1, and 7-10 corresponds to VT2.

EPOC

During aerobic exercise, the supply of oxygen does not always meet the need for oxygen, leaving the body with a deficit. Excess post-exercise oxygen consumption (EPOC) is the oxygen needed after a workout in order for the body to return to its resting state and temperature. The oxygen is used by the body to clear CO_2 from tissue, deplete lactic acid, restore adenosine triphosphate (ATP) levels, and increase blood oxygen levels. Because the use of oxygen burns calories (5 calories for every liter of oxygen), as many as 150 calories can be burned during EPOC (Anderson, 2015). This is important to remember as recovery time differs for clients with chronic disease, and exercise programming needs to be adjusted accordingly.

Discussion and application

1. Define lactate threshold and anaerobic threshold, and how they relate to RPE.
2. Assessing maximal cardiorespiratory capacity can be expensive, time consuming, and may require specialized personnel and equipment. Which assessment is best suited for your situation? Describe the procedure, and how you would explain the benefits to a client

References

American College of Sports Medicine. (2018). *ACSM's resources for the exercise physiologist: A practical guide for the health fitness professional* (P. Magyari, R. Lite, M. W. Kilpatrick, & J. E. Schoffstall Eds. 2 ed.). Philadelphia, PA: Wolters Kluwer.

American Council on Exercise. (n.d.). Key concept: Ventilatory threshold testing. Retrieved from https://acewebcontent.azureedge.net/certifiednews/images/article/pdfs/VT_Testing.pdf

Anderson, J. (2015). Burn it: Train to achieve afterburn. *American Fitness, 33*(2), 16-18. Retrieved from https://magazine.nasm.org/american-fitness-magazine/issues

Durstine, J. L., Painter, P., Franklin, B. A., Morgan, D., Pitetti, K. H., & Roberts, S. O. (2000). Physical activity for the chronically ill and disabled. *Sports Medicine, 30*(3), 207-219. https://doi.org/10.2165/00007256-200030030-00005

Galati, T. (2015). Applying the ACE Integrated Fitness Training model in the medical exercise setting in J.S. Skinner, C.X. Bryant, S. Merrill, & D.J. Green (Eds), *American Council on Exercise medical exercise specialist manual.* San Diego, CA: American Council on Exercise.

Garber, C. E., Blissmer, B., Deschenes, M. R., Franklin, B. A., Lamonte, M. J., Lee, I. M.,...Swain, D. P. (2011). Quantity and quality of exercise for developing and maintaining cardiorespiratory, musculoskeletal, and neuromotor fitness in apparently healthy adults: Guidance for prescribing exercise. *Medicine and Science in Sports and Exercise, 43*(7), 1334-1359. https://doi.org/10.1249/MSS.0b013e318213fefb

Mezzani, A., Hamm, L. F., Jones, A. M., McBride, P. E., Moholdt, T., Stone, J. A.,...Canadian Association of Cardiac, R. (2012). Aerobic exercise intensity assessment and prescription in cardiac rehabilitation: A joint position statement of the European Association for Cardiovascular Prevention and Rehabilitation, the American Association of Cardiovascular and Pulmonary Rehabilitation, and the Canadian Association of Cardiac Rehabilitation. *Journal of Cardiopulmonary Rehabilitation and Prevention, 32*(6), 327-350. https://doi.org/10.1097/HCR.0b013e3182757050

Noonan, V., & Dean, E. (2000). Submaximal exercise testing: Clinical application and interpretation. *Physical Therapy, 80*(8), 782-807. https://doi.org/10.1093/ptj/80.8.782

Scherr, J., Wolfarth, B., Christle, J. W., Pressler, A., Wagenpfeil, S., & Halle, M. (2013). Associations between Borg's rating of perceived exertion and physiological measures of exercise intensity. *European Journal of Applied Physiology, 113*(1), 147-155. https://org/10.1007/s00421-012-2421-x

Sartor, F., Bonomi, A. G., Kubis, H.-P., Vernillo, G., Torre, A. L., Veicsteinas, A., & Morree, H. M. d. (2013). Estimation of maximal oxygen uptake via submaximal exercise testing in sports, clinical, and home settings. *Sports Medicine, 43*(9), 865-873. https://doi.org/10.1007/s40279-013-0068-3

Woltmann, M. L., Foster, C., Porcari, J. P., Camic, C. L., Dodge, C., Haible, S., & Mikat, R. P. (2015). Evidence that the talk test can be used to regulate exercise intensity. *Journal of Strength and Conditioning Research, 29*(5), 1248-1254. https://doi.org/10.1519/JSC.0000000000000811

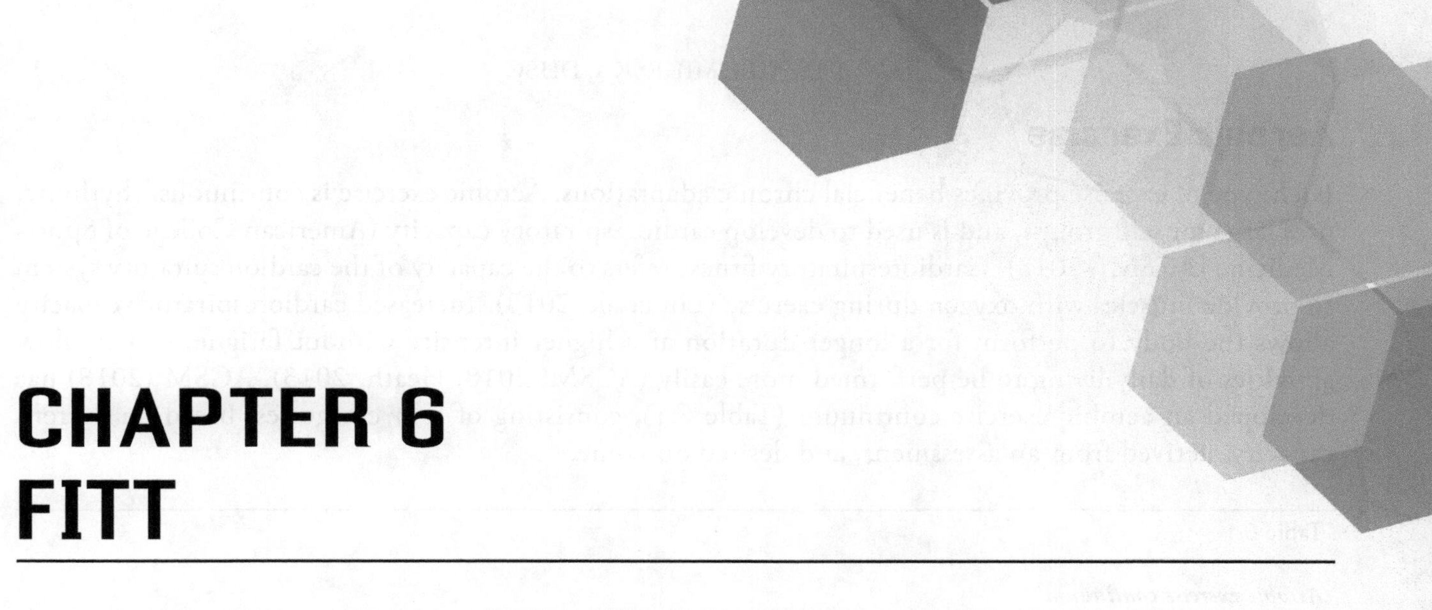

CHAPTER 6
FITT

By the end of this chapter you will understand:

- Components of fitness
- Frequency
- Intensity
- Time
- Type

Overall health is affected by each component of fitness (Garber et al., 2011). As fitness professionals, we may focus on one aspect, or mostly on one aspect. For example, maybe you are strength and conditioning coach, so your work revolves around athletes becoming stronger and faster, or maybe you are a yoga instructor who helps people with coordination and proprioception, or you are a running coach who trains individuals to run 26.2 miles. Regardless, some of this may, and should seem remedial, but it is worth reviewing to gain a deeper understanding, or simply as a reminder, of how it all connects.

The components of fitness are:

- Cardiorespiratory/Aerobic
- Muscular fitness
- Flexibility
- Neuromuscular fitness/Mind-body exercise
- Body composition (discussed in depth in Chapters 10 & 11)

Aerobic Exercise

Each type of exercise provides beneficial chronic adaptations. Aerobic exercise is continuous, rhythmic, uses large muscle groups, and is used to develop cardiorespiratory capacity (American College of Sports Medicine [ACSM], 2018). Cardiorespiratory fitness refers to the capacity of the cardiorespiratory system to provide muscles with oxygen during exercise (Lin et al., 2015). Increased cardiorespiratory capacity allows the body to perform for a longer duration at a higher intensity without fatigue; which allow activities of daily living to be performed more easily (ACSM, 2018; Heath, 2013). ACSM (2018) has developed an aerobic exercise continuum (Table 6.1), consisting of four categories, based on current capacity, derived from an assessment, and desired outcome.

Table 6.1

Aerobic exercise continuum

Level	Intensity	Examples
1	For deconditioned clients, requires minimal skill	Walking and aquatic exercise
2	Vigorous intensity exercise for currently active clients; requires minimal skill	Jogging/running, rowing, elliptical, and spinning
3	For moderately fit and skilled clients	Cross country skiing, skating, and swimming
4	Indicates a client can participate in recreational sports	Racquet sports, downhill skiing, or vigorous hiking

Chronic adaptations to aerobic exercise include increased cardiac output and stroke volume, reduced heart rate, and increased capillarization. Neural adaptions begin immediately and increase as a client progresses into skilled activity. Muscular endurance and power will increase in direct proportion to exercise intensity, as will bone growth, and tendon and ligament strength; the more intense the exercise, the greater the growth and strengthening (Swank, 2008). Similarly, there appears to be a dose-response relationship favoring the acute and chronic benefits of aerobic exercise on cardiometabolic risk factors, indicating regular exercise, as proposed in the frequency, intensity, time, and type (FITT) guidelines (Table 6.3), results in a long-term positive effect. Also, there is evidence suggesting cardiovascular disease (CVD) risk factors are mediated at capacities starting at one-half the recommended volume, and cardiorespiratory fitness may be a better predictor of CVD mortality and morbidity than smoking, hypertension, and diabetes (Garber et al., 2011; Kamil-Rosenberg & Garber, 2016).

Muscular Fitness

Muscular fitness refers to strength, power, and endurance.

- Muscular strength is the ability to exert force at a certain speed; force = mass x acceleration.
- Muscular power is the ability to exert force rapidly; power = force x velocity.
- Muscular endurance is the ability to perform repeated muscular contractions over time.

Although the dose-response relationship between muscular fitness and health outcomes is still under investigation, associated benefits of muscular fitness are increased functional capacity and neuromuscular control; improved cardiometabolic risk factor profiles, such as insulin resistance and blood pressure; a lower risk of CVD events and all-cause mortality; and a lower risk for nonfatal diseases (Garber et al., 2011; Heath, 2013). Additionally, there is an increase in enzyme activity, metabolic energy stores, connective tissue strength, and a decrease in body fat percentage (Ratamess, 2008). Weight bearing exercise has also been associated with increased bone mineral density, reduced incidence of osteoarthritis, improved energy levels, and reduced depression and anxiety. There are four commonly used types of resistance training (ACSM, 2018):

- Dynamic constant external resistance (DCER) refers to training in which a weight being lifted does not change. The original term, *isotonic* (same tension), is not an accurate description as the tension changes as muscle fibers lengthen, and joint length and angle vary throughout the range of motion (ROM). Free-weights, dumbbells, bodyweight, and some machines are examples of DCER.
- Due to the inconsistent tension in DCER, machines with cams and lever arms that ensure consistent tension throughout the ROM have been developed. These variable resistance machines change the resistant force to overcome the deficits in DCER by matching the strength curve. Accommodated resistance is a form of variable resistance training that uses bands and chains, in conjunction with free weighs, dumbbells, or body weight, to provide less resistance at the weakest part of the lift, and greater resistance as the lift continues through the ROM.
- Isokinetic (same speed) uses specially designed machines to keep the rate of the movement constant by changing the amount of resistance throughout the ROM. Isokinetic machines are mostly used in physical therapy and rehabilitation settings. However, by allowing an increase of movement speed, sports that require high velocity can also benefit from isokinetic training.
- Plyometric training improves neuromuscular performance by rapidly stretching a muscle (eccentric), immediately followed by rapidly shortening the muscle (concentric). Jumping, hopping, and medicine ball and rope slams are examples of plyometric training.

Table 6.3 details FITT guidelines for resistance training.

Flexibility

Flexibility refers to the range of motion (ROM) of a joint or body segment. ROM can be determined by the type of joint, properties of muscles, ligaments, and tendons interacting with a joint, level of activity, age, and gender (ACSM, 2018; Jeffreys, 2008). Proper ROM can help reduce injuries and increase physical performance. Conversely, limited ROM, or short, tight muscles will not contract or relax efficiently, altering the length-tension and force-couple relationships, resulting in a decrease of strength and adequate circulation. More importantly, the altered muscular relationships will decrease mobility resulting in poor posture, limited functional capacity, and impair activities of daily living (ADLs). Table 6.2 details the average ROM for healthy adults.

Table 6.2

Average range of motion for healthy adults

Joint and movement	Range of motion	Joint and movement	Range of motion	Joint and movement	Range of motion
Hip		Shoulder/Scapulae		Cervical spine	
Flexion	100-120	Flexion	150-180	Flexion	45-50
Extension	10-30	Extension	50-60	Extension	45-75
Abduction	40-45	Abduction	180	Lateral flexion	45
Adduction	20-30	Internal rotation	70-80	Rotation	65-75
Internal rotation	35-45	External rotation	90	Thoracic Spine	
External rotation	45-60	Horizontal adduction	90	Flexion	30-40
Knee		Horizontal Abduction	30-40	Extension	20-30
Flexion	125-145	Elbow		Lateral flexion	120-25
Extension	0-10	Flexion	145	Rotation	35
Ankle		Extension	0	Lumbar Spine	
Dorsiflexion	20	Radio-ulnar		Flexion	40-45
Plantarflexion	45-50	Pronation	90	Extension	30-40
Subtalar		Supination	90	Lateral flexion	20
Inversion	30-35	Wrist		Rotation	10-15
Eversion	15-20	Flexion	80		
		Extension	70		
		Radial deviation	20		
		Ulnar deviation	45		

Comana & McGrath, 2015; Soucie et al., 2011

There are a number of modes of flexibility (ACSM, 2018; Behm, Blazevich, Kay, & McHugh, 2016; Bushman, 2016; Jeffreys, 2008; Keteyian, 2013):

- Static stretching (SS) is often referred to as *stretch and hold* and may be the most common stretching due to the ease of implementation. SS involves lengthening a muscle until the point of discomfort, and then holding the position for a prescribed time; usually 20-30 seconds, but often up to 60 seconds for deconditioned adults. Although SS has been demonstrated to decrease muscle and joint stiffness, and increase ROM, there is some evidence, because of the slow and controlled nature, it may hinder sports performance when performed prior to an event.
- Active and passive stretching are similar to SS in that a muscle is lengthened and then held. However active stretching uses an antagonist muscle or muscle group to hold the stretch, and passive stretching uses an aid such as a yoga band or a partner to assist.
- Dynamic stretching (DS) increases ROM by slowly and repeatedly moving through a specific movement or pattern around an active joint or body segment. DS has become increasingly popular prior to activity and athletic events as it increases core temperature, muscle compliance, and nerve conduction. Additionally, the design of DS movements is limited only by imagination and mechanical dysfunction.

- Proprioceptive Neuromuscular Facilitation (PNF) stretching, is also known as *contract and relax stretching*. It is performed by contracting a muscle, using isometrics or against a resistant force, followed by SS. Through the reciprocal inhibition response of the Golgi tendon organs, a muscle and tendons elongate to achieve a greater ROM than SS alone. It is not as popular as other forms of flexibility, as it is difficult to perform alone, and although popular with physical therapists due to the controlled nature, PNF is becoming more prominent in athletics.
- Ballistic stretching uses repetitive rapid or bobbing movements to quickly move a muscle into an elongated position, followed quickly by relaxation of the muscle. Ballistic stretching is often used as a pre-exercise warm-up and prior to athletic events. However, due to the fast nature of the movement, the stretch reflex is activated but the muscle does not have time to respond, creating an opportunity for injury to the muscle or connective tissue.

Table 6.3 details FITT recommendations for stretching and flexibility.

Neuromuscular Fitness

Neuromuscular fitness, also known as mind-body exercise, can in part, be defined as exercise that integrates the brain, mind, body, and behavior, and promotes flexibility, strength, and relaxation (Kenney & Alexander, 2015; Rudaz, Ledermann, & Witt, 2017). Neuromuscular exercise has been demonstrated to better manage CVD, diabetes, and hypertension (La Forge, 2009). Although any exercise can incorporate or increase the mind-body connection, yoga and Tai-chi are traditionally thought of as mind-body modalities, and more recently Pilates (La Forge, 2015). To be considered as a form of neuromuscular fitness, the exercise should (La Forge, 2016):

- Be non-competitive and meditative.
- Include low- to moderate-level muscular activity that increases proprioceptive awareness.
- Include breath-centering techniques.
- Incorporate proper anatomical alignment in any static position or movement patterns.
- Be energy-centric and encourage awareness of the movement and flow.

Table 6.3 details FITT recommendations for neuromuscular exercise.

FITT guidelines need to be considered for the mode of exercise, each client, and the specific circumstances; all based on assessments. To achieve results, a minimum intensity threshold must be realized; therefore, the proposed guidelines are based on the overload principle of training to challenge physiological parameters. Table 6.3 details the current FITT recommendations.

Table 6.3

FITT guidelines

Mode	Frequency	Intensity	Time	Type
Cardiorespiratory Exercise/ Aerobic	≥ 5 days/week of moderate intensity or ≥ 3 days/ week of vigorous intensity	Moderate or vigorous	30-60 min/day of moderate (150 min/ week) 20-60 min/day of vigorous (75 min/ week)	Continuous, rhythmic, includes all major muscle groups
Older or deconditioned individuals		Light to moderate	bouts of <10 min can be beneficial	
Resistance Exercise	Each major muscle group 2-3 days/ week	60%–70% of the 1RM (moderate to hard intensity) for novice to intermediate exercisers ≥80% of the 1RM (hard to very hard intensity) for experienced strength trainers <50% of the 1RM for muscular endurance	8–12 reps to improve strength 15–20 reps to improve muscular endurance 2-4 sets	Resistance exercises involving each major muscle group, targeting larger groups first
Older or deconditioned individuals		Light intensity; 40-50% 1RM	10–15 reps for strength 15-20 reps for muscular endurance A single set can be effective	
Posture Restoration	1-2x/day	Small overload in controlled positions	Hold isometric contractions for 5-10 seconds Dynamic contractions: 1-2 sets, 12-20 reps	30-45 minutes 1-3 months
Flexibility	≥ 2-3 days/week	Stretch to the point of feeling tightness or slight discomfort	Static stretching hold for 10-30 sec. or up to 60 sec. for older individuals For PNF stretching, a 3- to 6-sec contraction at 20%–75% maximum voluntary contraction followed by a 10-30 sec. assisted stretch	Static flexibility, Dynamic flexibility PNF

Older or deconditioned individuals			Static stretching hold for up to 60 sec.	
Posture Restoration	10 min bouts 1-2x/day	Static-to the point of tension Dynamic-controlled to the point of resistance	Static—2-4 reps; 30-60 seconds Dynamic—1-2 sets, 5-10 reps	30-45 min 1-3 months
Neuromuscular exercise training The effectiveness of neuromuscular exercise training in younger and middle-aged persons has not been Established	≥2-3 days/week	N/A	≥20-30 min/bout	Exercise that challenges motor skills, coordination, and proprioception such as Yoga or Tai Chi

ACSM, 2018; Garber et al., 2011

Discussion and application

1. Outline the components of FITT as they pertain to flexibility, cardiovascular exercise, and resistance training.
2. Define joint stability and joint mobility, and how will you explain the importance of each to a client?

References

American College of Sports Medicine. (2018). *ACSM's resources for the exercise physiologist: A practical guide for the health fitness professional* (P. Magyari, R. Lite, M. W. Kilpatrick, & J. E. Schoffstall Eds. 2 ed.). Philadelphia, PA: Wolters Kluwer.

Behm, D. G., Blazevich, A. J., Kay, A. D., & McHugh, M. (2016). Acute effects of muscle stretching on physical performance, range of motion, and injury incidence in healthy active individuals: a systematic review. *Applied Physiology, Nutrition, and Metabolism, 41*(1), 1-11. https://doi.org/10.1139/apnm-2015-0235

Bushman, B. A. (2016). Flexibility Exercises and Performance. *ACSM's Health & Fitness Journal, 20*(5), 5-9. https://doi.org/10.1249/FIT.0000000000000226

Comana, F. & McGrath, C. (2015). Posture and movement in J.S. Skinner, C.X. Bryant, S. Merrill, & D.J. Green (Eds), *American Council on Exercise medical exercise specialist manual.* San Diego, CA: American Council on Exercise.

Garber, C. E., Blissmer, B., Deschenes, M. R., Franklin, B. A., Lamonte, M. J., Lee, I. M.,…Swain, D. P. (2011). Quantity and quality of exercise for developing and maintaining cardiorespiratory, musculoskeletal, and neuromotor fitness in apparently healthy adults: Guidance for prescribing exercise. *Medicine & Science in Sports & Exercise, 43*(7), 1334-1359. https://doi.org/10.1249/MSS.0b013e318213fefb

Heath, G.W. (2013). Behavioral approaches to physical activity promotion in J.K. Ehrman, P.M. Gordon, & P.S. Visich (Eds), *Clinical exercise physiology* (3rd Ed.). Champaign IL: Human Kinetics.

Jeffreys, I. (2008). Warm up and stretching in T.R. Baechle & R.W. Earle (Eds), *Essentials of strength training and conditioning* (3rd Ed.). Champaign, IL: Human Kinetics.

Kamil-Rosenberg, S., & Garber, C. E. (2016). Cardiac conditioning for healthy individuals: primary prevention of heart disease. *Current Physical Medicine and Rehabilitation Reports, 4*(3), 223-232. https://doi.org/10.1007/s40141-016-0130-9

Kenney, W. L. & Alexander, L. M. (2015). Hypertension in J.S. Skinner, C.X. Bryant, S. Merrill, & D.J. Green (Eds), *American Council on Exercise medical exercise specialist manual.* San Diego, CA: American Council on Exercise.

Keteyian, S. J. (2013). Graded exercise testing and exercise prescription in J.K. Ehrman, P.M. Gordon, & P.S. Visich (Eds), *Clinical exercise physiology* (3rd Ed.). Champaign IL: Human Kinetics.

Swank, A. (2008). Adaptations to aerobic endurance training programs in T.R. Baechle & R.W. Earle (Eds), *Essentials of strength training and conditioning* (3rd Ed.). Champaign, IL: Human Kinetics.

Ratamess, N.A. (2008). Adaptations to anaerobic training programs in T.R. Baechle & R.W. Earle (Eds), *Essentials of strength training and conditioning* (3rd Ed.). Champaign, IL: Human Kinetics.

La Forge, R. (2009). Mindful exercise and chronic disease. *IDEA Fitness Journal*, 72-75. Retrieved from https://www.ideafit.com/fitness-library/mindful-exercise-and-chronic-disease

La Forge, R. (2015). Coronary heart disease in J.S. Skinner, C.X. Bryant, S. Merrill, & D.J. Green (Eds), *American Council on Exercise medical exercise specialist manual.* San Diego, CA: American Council on Exercise.

La Forge, R. (2016). Mind-body (mindful) exercise in practice. *ACSM's Health & Fitness Journal, 20*(4), 6-8. Retrieved from https://journals.lww.com/acsm-healthfitness/pages/default.aspx

Lin, X., Zhang, X., Guo, J., Roberts, C. K., McKenzie, S., Wu, W. C.,…Song, Y. (2015). Effects of exercise training on cardiorespiratory fitness and biomarkers of cardiometabolic health: A systematic review and meta-analysis of randomized controlled trials. *Journal of the American Heart Association*, 4(7). https://doi.org/10.1161/JAHA.115.002014

Rudaz, M., Ledermann, T., & Witt, C. M. (2017). Mind-body medicine and the treatment of chronic illnesses. *Swiss Sports & Exercise Medicine, 65*(2), 26-30. https://doi.org/10.5167/uzh-148692

Soucie, J. M., Wang, C., Forsyth, A., Funk, S., Denny, M., Roach, K. E.,…Hemophilia Treatment Center Network. (2011). Range of motion measurements: Reference values and a database for comparison studies. *Haemophilia, 17*(3), 500-507. https://doi.org/10.1111/j.1365-2516.2010.02399.x

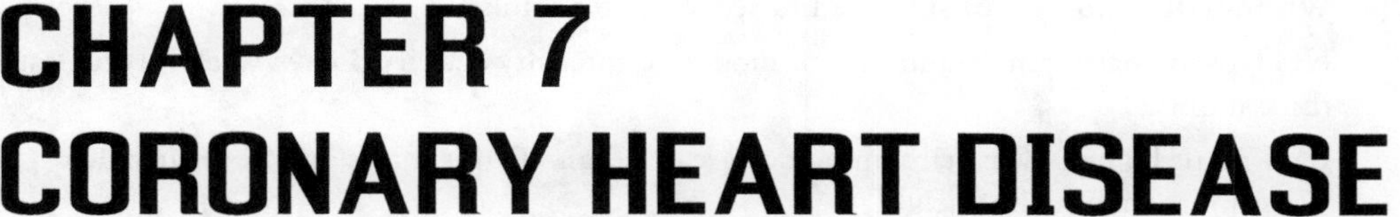

CHAPTER 7
CORONARY HEART DISEASE

By the end of this chapter you will understand:

- Background
- Risk factors
- Pre-participation health screening
- Contraindications
- Exercise recommendations
- Nutrition guidelines

Background

Cardiovascular disease (CVD) accounts for more than 17 million annual deaths worldwide and close to 800,000 in the U.S. (Kachur, et al., 2017). Coronary heart disease (CHD), a subset of CVD, occurs when the small blood vessels leading to the heart narrow, preventing blood and oxygen from passing. In the U.S., 1.5 million people suffer from CHD, and CHD accounts for almost 500,000 deaths annually (Kamil-Rosenberg, & Garber, 2016). Due to the prevalence of CVD, it is important for a CXS to recognize the risk factors and know which clients may be at risk. Table 7.1 details CVD risk factors.

Table 7.1

CVD risk factors

Positive Risk Factor	Criteria
Age	Males -45 or older; Females 55 or older
Family History	Heart attack, coronary revascularization, or sudden death. First degree relative: Male prior to 55 or female prior to 65 years of age
Cigarette Smoking	Within last 6 months, or subjected to second hand smoke
Sedentary Lifestyle	NOT participating in 30 minutes of moderate-intensity activity 3 days/week for the last three months
Obesity	BMI 30 or higher. Waist circumference greater than 40" for males or 35" for females. Waist more than half of height.
Hypertension	BP greater than 139/89, or currently on antihypertension medication.
Dyslipidemia (Cholesterol)	LDL greater than 129, HDL less than 40, total greater than 200, or currently on medication
Pre-Diabetes/Diabetes	Fasting glucose greater than 99
Negative Risk Factor	Criteria
High Serum HDL	HDL greater than 60

CHD is the result of atherosclerosis. Atherosclerosis occurs when the inner walls of blood vessels lose elasticity, and become hard and thick, from accumulated plaque from an excess of lipoproteins in the blood. The most common symptom of CHD is a myocardial infarction (MI), or heart attack (La Forge, 2015), and occurs when the plaque lining the walls of blood vessels breaks free and enters the heart. The most common symptoms of an MI are shortness of breath, syncope, nausea, and diffuse (rather than localized) pain. Another indication of CHD is angina pectoris. Angina pectoris, also associated with narrowing of blood vessel walls, is discomfort in the chest, arms, shoulder, and jaw. Unstable angina requires immediate medical attention however, a CXS can work with clients who have predictable, or stable angina. Stable angina can be categorized into the activity or functional, classifications listed below (La Forge, 2015).

- Class I angina indicates ordinary physical activity does not provoke symptoms, but rapid, prolonged exertion may cause chest pain.
- Class II angina is a slight limitation in physical activity.
- Class III angina is a severe limitation in physical activity.
- Class IV angina is a complete inability to perform physical activity without discomfort.

Heart failure occurs when cardiac output does not meet the metabolic demands of the body, and cardiac dysrhythmia occurs when there is a disruption in the beating rhythm of the heart. Heart failure and cardiac dysrhythmia are often the result of a MI; whereas unstable angina may proceed a MI.

Pre-participation Health Screening

The first line of treatment following a CHD event is cardiac rehabilitation, focused on exercise, lifestyle adaptations, and nutrition counseling. Ideally, a client who has experienced a CHD event will have completed early phase cardiac rehabilitation (24–36 sessions) prior to an exercise program with a CXS

(Kachur, et al., 2017; La Forge 2015). A CXS can work with clients at risk for CHD, but asymptomatic or who have stable CHD and are medically cleared for exercise.

Although discussed in Chapter 2, it is worth repeating, the American College of Sports Medicine (ACSM) has new pre-participation health screening recommendations (Magal & Riebe, 2016). Exercise is safe for most people, and the absolute risk of a cardiovascular event is extremely low (Magal & Riebe, 2016). It is thought previous guidelines were too conservative, requiring up to 95% of clients, age 40 and over to seek medical clearance prior to beginning an exercise program; consequently, discouraging many from ever starting.

Just to reiterate, the objective of the new guidelines are similar to previous guidelines (Magal & Riebe, 2016):

1. To identify individuals who should receive medical clearance before starting a new program or increasing the frequency, intensity, and/or volume of an existing exercise program.
2. To identify individuals who present with CV, metabolic, and/or renal diseases and will benefit from participating in a medically-supervised exercise program.
3. To identify individuals with CV, metabolic, and/or renal diseases who must wait until their medical condition(s) have improved to proceed with an exercise program.

A sample Physical Activity Risk Stratification form can be found in Appendix A.

Contraindications

In addition to the CVD risk factors listed in Table 7.1, the following are common, absolute contraindications to exercise training for clients with CHD (ACSM, 2018; Gielen, Laughlin, O'Conner, & Duncker, 2015; Kachur et al., 2017; La Forge, 2015).

- Unstable angina
- Severe or symptomatic aortic stenosis
- Decompensated heart failure—new or worsening signs and symptoms of HF
- Severe obstructive cardiomyopathy
- Acute cardiac mural thrombus—ventricle wall clot
- Acute deep venous thrombus
- Recent embolism
- Recent myocardial infarction
- Uncontrolled cardiac arrhythmia
- Uncompensated symptomatic CHF
- Acute myocarditis or pericarditis
- Uncontrolled HTN (resting SBP >180 mm Hg and/or resting DBP >110 mm Hg)
- Orthostatic BP drop of >20 mm Hg

- Uncontrolled sinus tachycardia
- Thrombophlebitis
- Illness or fever

Exercise Recommendations

For a client with CHD, the clearance for exercise can only be made by a physician and is outside the scope of practice of a CXS. However, it should be noted some contraindications can be considered relative; meaning the benefits of exercise can outweigh the risks, and a client should be allowed to proceed with caution (ACSM, 2018; Gielen et al., 2015). Accordingly, a training session should end at the first sign of symptoms, and resume only after the symptoms have been resolved. Some relative contraindications to exercise for clients with CHD are stable angina, controlled hypertension, asymptomatic tachyarrhythmia and bradyarrhythmia, and uncorrected anemia (Gielen et al., 2015). FITT Guidelines for clients with stable CHD are in Table 7.2.

Table 7.2

FITT Guidelines for clients with stable coronary heart disease

	Frequency	Intensity	Time	Type	Caution
Aerobic	3-7 days/ week 3 days if all bouts are vigorous	Initial Stage: 30-55% HRR Deconditioned or at-risk: 30-39% HRR Stable CHD: Moderate—40-60% HRR or RPE <11-14 Vigorous—60-90% HRR	Deconditioned or at-risk: 1-10 min bouts, 3x/ day Stable CHD: 20-60 min/session or 2000 kcal expenditure/week	Rhythmic motion using large muscle groups	Start slow, and warm up gradually. Limit heavy weights to avoid breath holding, isometric exercise, muscular contraction failure, and Valsalva maneuver.
Resistance Training	2-3 days/ week	General: 60-80% 1RM (low-moderate) Deconditioned or at-risk: <40% 1RM	General: 8-12 exercises 1-4 sets Deconditioned or at-risk: 10-15 reps 1 set	Bands, light hand weights, machines.	Avoid rapid changes in body position Monitor the client for a few minutes after the exercise has ended

ACSM, 2018; Kamil-Rosenberg & Garber, 2016; La Forge, 2015

Nutrition Basics

Although a CXS is not qualified to provide nutrition guidance to a client (unless a CXS has formal training in nutrition such as a registered dietician), there are recommendations that can be discussed. The primary cause for CHD is atherosclerosis, a hardening and narrowing of blood vessels due to fatty plaque build-up. Low-density lipoproteins (LDL) contribute to atherosclerosis; therefore, a main goal of any diet should be to reduce LDL cholesterol. Omega-3 fatty acids have been associated with a reduction of arrhythmias and the progression of atherosclerosis. Plant sterols and stanols mimic cholesterol and may reduce cholesterol uptake. Conservative alcohol consumption (1-2 drinks/day) can reduce blood pressure by relaxing the endothelial cells that line blood vessel walls, and 25-30 grams of fiber daily can aid in the reduction of total and LDL cholesterol.

Discussion and application

1. Describe the differences between angina pectoris, myocardial infarction, and heart failure.
2. Describe some contraindications to exercise training for client experiencing CHD.

References

American College of Sports Medicine. (2018). *ACSM's resources for the exercise physiologist: A practical guide for the health fitness professional* (P. Magyari, R. Lite, M. W. Kilpatrick, & J. E. Schoffstall Eds. 2 ed.). Philadelphia, PA: Wolters Kluwer.

Gielen, S., Laughlin, M. H., O'Conner, C., & Duncker, D. J. (2015). Exercise training in patients with heart disease: Review of beneficial effects and clinical recommendations. *Progress in Cardiovascular Disease, 57*(4), 347-355. https://doi.org/10.1016/j.pcad.2014.10.001

Kachur, S., Chongthammakun, V., Lavie, C. J., De Schutter, A., Arena, R., Milani, R. V., & Franklin, B. A. (2017). Impact of cardiac rehabilitation and exercise training programs in coronary heart disease. *Progress in Cardiovascular Disease, 60*(1), 103-114. https://doi.org/10.1016/j.pcad.2017.07.002

Kamil-Rosenberg, S., & Garber, C. E. (2016). Cardiac conditioning for healthy individuals: Primary prevention of heart disease. *Current Physical Medicine and Rehabilitation Reports, 4*(3), 223-232. https://doi.org/10.1007/s40141-016-0130-9

La Forge, R. (2015). Coronary heart disease in J.S. Skinner, C.X. Bryant, S. Merrill, & D.J. Green (Eds), *American Council on Exercise medical exercise specialist manual.* San Diego, CA: American Council on Exercise.

Magal, M., & Riebe, D. (2016). New preparticipation health screening: What exercise professionals need to know. *ACSM's Health & Fitness Journal, 20*(3), 22-27. https://doi.org/10.1249/FIT.0000000000000202

CHAPTER 8
HYPERTENSION

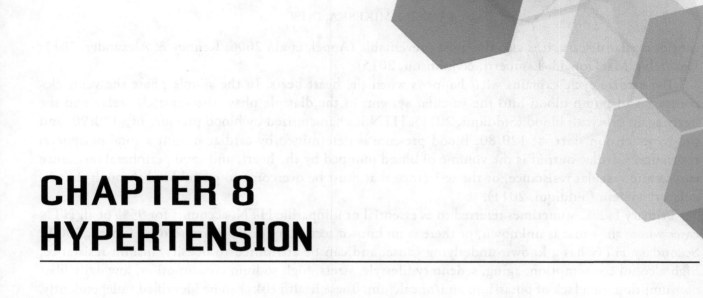

By the end of this chapter you will understand:

- Hypertension and comorbidities
    - o Prevalence
    - o Risk factors
- Characteristics of prehypertension and hypertension
- Current guidelines and recommendations
    - o Pharmacology
    - o Activity
        - ▪ Precautions
        - ▪ Contraindications
        - ▪ Nutrition

Characteristics

Hypertension (HTN) and prehypertension affect over 160 million U.S. adults, and nearly a billion individuals worldwide. HTN is an independent risk factor for coronary artery disease, stroke, renal failure, heart failure, atrial fibrillation, valvular disease, sudden cardiac death, cardiomyopathy, and aortic aneurysms (Appel et al., 2006). Accordingly, the higher the blood pressure, the greater the risk for a cardiovascualr event, kidney failure, or stroke (Carretero & Oparil, 2000; Kenney & Alexander, 2015; Kokubo & Matsumoto, 2016). HTN is the most common chronic disease risk factor; adults over 50 years of age have close to a 90% chance of developing HTN; it is the costliest risk factor for cardiovascular disease; it is also the most preventable (Appel, et al., 2006; Kenney & Alexander, 2015; Pescatello, MacDonald, Lamberti, & Johnson, 2015).

The cardiac cycle explains what happens when the heart beats. In the systole phase the ventricles contract and pump blood into the vascular system; in the diastole phase the ventricles relax and the heart again fills with blood (Siddiqui, 2011). HTN is characterized by blood pressure of≥140/90, and pre-hypertension starts at 120/80. Blood pressure is determined by cardiac output x total peripheral resistance. Cardiac output is the volume of blood pumped by the heart, and total peripheral resistance is systemic vascular resistance, or the resistance that must be overcome to push blood through the circulatory system (Siddiqui, 2011).

Primary HTN, sometimes referred to as essential or idiopathic HTN, accounts for 95% of all HTN cases where the cause is unknown, or there is no known secondary cause (Carretero, & Oparil, 2000). Secondary HTN has a known underlying cause, and can be attributed to obesity, insulin resistance, high alcohol consumption, aging, sedentary lifestyle, stress, high sodium consumption, low daily fiber consumption, or a lack of potassium and/or calcium. These health risks can be identified independently, but are often found in combinations.

Pharmacological Therapy

It is important for a CXS to know the medications a client is prescribed as many common medications used to treat HTN have side effects and may also affect exercise performance. Use, mechanisms, and side effects of common HTN medications are listed in Table 8.1.

Table 8.1

Hypertension medications and side effects

Drug	Mechanism	Side effects	Consideration
Beta Blockers	Blocks beta receptors	Stunts HR May stunt symptoms of hypoglycemia May cause dizziness or fatigue	Measure exercise intensity via RPE rather than HR
Diuretics	Reduces extra-cellular fluid	Dehydration May decrease exercise capacity May cause confusion or weakness	Hydrate. Hydrate, Hydrate
ACE inhibitors and ARBs	Vasodilation	None that effect exercise	May cause hypotension
Calcium channel blockers	Blocks calcium from entering cardiac muscle	Stunts HR May cause orthostatic hypotension, headaches, and dizziness	Measure exercise intensity via RPE rather than HR Stand up carefully and slowly
Angiotensin Receptor Blocker	Blocks angiotensin receptors	Stunts HR May cause orthostatic hypotension, headaches, and dizziness	Measure exercise intensity via RPE rather than HR Stand up carefully and slowly

American College of Sports Medicine [ACSM], 2018; Kenney & Alexander, 2015; Swank & Sharp, 2018

Exercise Training

Due to a reduction in peripheral vascular resistance, exercise training and a high level of fitness are associated with lower levels of HTN. It has been estimated for a 10% weight gain, there is a 6.5 mm Hg increase in systolic BP. Because of the deleterious effects of weight on BP, clients should work toward an expenditure of 2000 kcal/week with a focus on aerobic exercise. For adults with HTN, aerobic exercise training lowers blood pressure 5–7 mmHg, while resistance training lowers blood pressure 2–3 mmHg (Carretero & Oparil, 2000; Pescatello et al., 2015). Due to post-exercise hypotension, it is recommended clients with HTN perform aerobic exercise on most days of the week with an intensity of 40-60% HRR or an RPE of 11-13. Because aerobic training lowers BP to a greater extent than resistance training, resistance training should be used as adjunct to aerobic training and performed 2-3 days per week at an intensity of 60-80% 1RM. Because of the combination of light weights and fast pace, high intensity interval training should also be considered. FITT recommendations for clients with HTN are detailed in Table 8.2.

Similar to CHD, a CXS should not work with clients who have uncontrolled HTN.

Table 8.2

FITT recommendations for hypertension

Controlled HTN	Frequency	Intensity	Time	Type
Aerobic	Preferably all days of the week	Most clients should perform at a moderate intensity: 40-60% HRR RPE of 11-13 Vigorous: 60-80% HRR RPE of 14-16	Most people: 30-60 Min Deconditioned or at-risk: 1-10 min bouts, 3x/day	Rhythmic motion using large muscle groups.
Resistance Training	2-3 days/ week with at least 48 hours between bouts	60-70% 1RM (low-moderate) Progress to 80% 1RM Novice and beginners start at 40-50% 1RM	8-12 reps A minimum of one set. 1-4 sets 8-10 exercises (all of major muscle groups) No less than 20 minutes per session	Free weights and machines Avoid the Valsalva maneuver
Flexibility	2-3 days/ week	Slight discomfort or mild tightness	Static stretch each major muscle group 2-4 reps 10-30 seconds 10 minutes each session	Static Dynamic PNF
Neuromuscular	2-3 days/ week	Low to moderate	20-30 minutes	Yoga Pilates Tai Chi Involve all major muscle groups, using functional movement patterns and flexibility exercises to increase motor skills.

Combined Ideal	Everyday	Low, moderate, or vigorous, with an emphasis on moderate	20-30 minutes/day Total of 90->150 minutes/week	Combine all types, with an emphasis on aerobic and resistance with flexibility and neuromuscular added in.

ACSM, 2018; Kenney & Alexander, 2015; Pescatello, et al., 2015; Pescatello, 2019; Swank & Sharp, 2018

Caution

It is possible, in clients with HTN, that an increase in arterial blood pressure may dislodge arterial plaque causing a myocardial infarction or stroke. Further, any existing endothelial damage may be exacerbated (ACSM, 2018). Because of a reduction in skin blood flow, clients with HTN may not be able to dissipate heat effectively, disrupting normal thermoregulation (Kenney & Alexander, 2015). Therefore, exercise load needs to be carefully monitored and modified, or ended at the first sign of heat stress. Also, keep in mind, beta-blockers blunt the normal heart rate response nullifying the recommendation of 40-60% HHR, and the RPE scale will have to be used to gauge exercise intensity.

Contraindications and indications for stopping exercise include:

- Onset of angina
- Failure of HR to increase with intensity
- A drop in SBP of ≥10 with an increase in intensity
- A change in heart rhythm
- A rise of SBP > 250 or DBP >115
- Shortness of breath
- Leg cramps or claudication
- Light headedness or confusion
- Pallor or cold and clammy skin
- Nausea
- Signs of severe fatigue

Nutritional Considerations

Although specific meal planning is the responsibility of a registered dietitian, nutrition basics can be discussed as they may affect some aspects of exercise. The list provides general guidelines for clients who suffer from HTN (Appell et al., 2006; Carretero & Oparil, 2000; Kenney & Alexander, 2015; Van Horn et al., 2016).

Keep in mind, it is outside the scope of practice of a CXS to provide nutrition counseling.

- Sodium levels should be kept to 2400mg/day for the general population, and no more than 1500mg/day for individuals suffering from HTN.
- The recommended intake for fiber is 28–30 gm/day.
- The recommended intake for potassium is 4700 mg/day.
- The recommended intake for calcium is 1000-1300 mg/day.
- Fruits and vegetables provide other vitamins and minerals; therefore increasing the consumption of fruits and vegetables is preferable over taking supplements.

Discussion and application

1. Discuss the benefits and concerns of exercise as it relates to HTN.
2. Using FITT, design an exercise program for a client with controlled HTN and explain your decisions

References

American College of Sports Medicine. (2018). ACSM's resources for the exercise physiologist: *A practical guide for the health fitness professional* (P. Magyari, R. Lite, M. W. Kilpatrick, & J. E. Schoffstall Eds. 2 ed.). Philadelphia, PA: Wolters Kluwer.

Appel, L. J., Brands, M. W., Daniels, S. R., Karanja, N., Elmer, P. J., Sacks, F. M., & American Heart Association. (2006). Dietary approaches to prevent and treat hypertension: A scientific statement from the American Heart Association. *Hypertension, 47*(2), 296-308. https://doi.org/10.1161/01.HYP.0000202568.01167.B6

Carretero, O. A., & Oparil, S. (2000). Essential hypertension part I: Definition and etiology. *Circulation*, (101), 329-335. http://dx.doi.org/10.1161/01.CIR.101.3.329

Kenney, W. L. & Alexander, L. M. (2015). Hypertension in J.S. Skinner, C.X. Bryant, S. Merrill, & D.J. Green (Eds), *American Council on Exercise medical exercise specialist manual.* San Diego, CA: American Council on Exercise.

Kokubo, Y., & Matsumoto, C. (2016). Hypertension is a risk factor for several types of heart disease: Review of prospective studies. In *Hypertension: From basic research to clinical practice* (pp. 419-426). Champaign, IL: Springer.

Pescatello, L. S., MacDonald, H. V., Lamberti, L., & Johnson, B. T. (2015). Exercise for hypertension: A prescription update integrating existing recommendations with emerging research. *Current Hypertension Reports, 17*(11), 87. https://doi.org/10.1007/s11906-015-0600-y

Pescatello, L. S. (2019). What's new in the ACSM pronouncement on exercise and hypertension? Retrieved from http://www.acsm.org/all-blog-posts/acsm-blog/acsm-blog/2019/06/11/new-acsm-pronouncement-exercise-hypertension

Siddiqui, A. (2011). Effects of vasodilation and arterial resistance on cardiac output. *Journal of Clinical & Experimental Cardiology, 02*(11). https://doi.org/10.4172/2155-9880.1000170

Swank, A. M. & Sharp, C. (2018). Cardiovascular conditions and disorders in P.L. Jacobs (Ed) *NSCA's essentials of training special populations.* Champaign, IL: Human Kinetics

Van Horn, L., Carson, J. A., Appel, L. J., Burke, L. E., Economos, C., Karmally, W.,...Stroke, C. (2016). Recommended dietary pattern to achieve adherence to the American Heart Association/American College of Cardiology (AHA/ACC) Guidelines: A scientific statement from the American Heart Association. *Circulation, 134*(22), e505-e529. https://doi.org/10.1161/CIR.0000000000000462

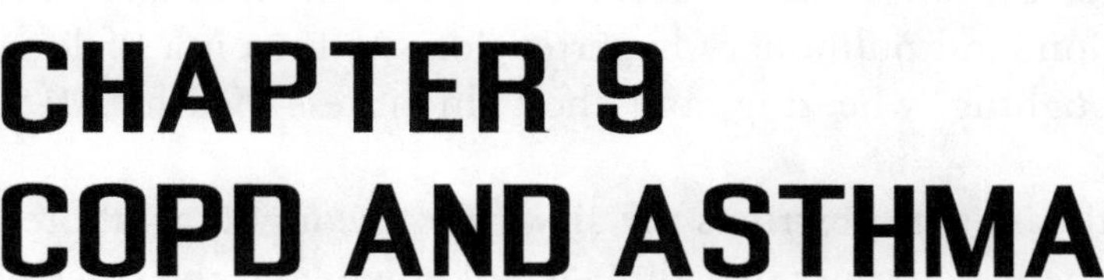

CHAPTER 9
COPD AND ASTHMA

By the end of this chapter you will understand:

- Characteristics and diagnostic criteria
    - o Chronic Obstructive Pulmonary Disorder
        - Bronchitis and emphysema
        - Asthma
- Statistics
- Treatment strategies
    - o Pharmacological
    - o Nutrition
    - o Exercise
        - Exercise induced asthma
        - FITT
- Risks and considerations

Chronic Obstructive Pulmonary Disorder

Chronic Obstructive Pulmonary Disorder (COPD) is a common preventable and treatable disease characterized by persistent, limited airflow that is usually progressive and irreversible. COPD is associated with an enhanced chronic inflammatory response in the airways and the lungs to noxious particles or gases, and exacerbations and comorbidities contribute to the overall severity in individual patients

(Global Initiative for Chronic Obstructive Lung Disease [GOLD], 2016). Bronchitis and emphysema are forms of COPD; and asthma can be present with or without COPD (American College of Sports Medicine [ACSM], 2018; GOLD, 2016).

Bronchitis is characterized by a sputum producing cough that is persistent for 3+ months, for 2 or more consecutive years (ACSM, 2018; GOLD, 2016). Chronic bronchitis can result in pulmonary inflammation that may damage the bronchial lining and obstruct airflow. Emphysema is characterized by the destruction of alveoli that causes poor gas exchange and an accumulation of air in lung tissue, often resulting in increased pulmonary circulation, and pulmonary hypertension. Asthma is a lifelong disease characterized by airflow obstruction, coughing, wheezing, and chest thightness (Muth, 2015; Silkoff et al., 2015).

Chronic asthma is a diverse inflammatory disease that obstructs the airway with coughing, labored breathing, and wheezing (Silkoff et al., 2015). The initial cause of asthma is unknown, and the severity of asthma is variable and may worsen or become better over time (Muth, 2015). There is a link between asthma and allergies, and accordingly, an asthma attack can be triggered by cold air, infections, animal dander or hair, dust mites, smoke, pollen, mold, stress, or exercise. Unfortunately, because the inflammatory pathways may vary between patients, the effectiveness of treatment plans also varies from patient to patient.

Statistics

In 2015, it was estimated over 65 million people worldwide suffered from COPD and 3.2 million people died. In the United States, COPD is the third leading cause of death due to disease, and it is estimated 16-24 million people have COPD (Krucik, 2018; Rundell, Smoliga, & Weiss, 2018). Although smoking is the leading cause of COPD, harmful pollutants such as chemicals, exhaust, dust, and secondhand smoke can also lead to COPD. The chronic airflow obstruction caused by COPD can lead to reduced cardiac function and hinder gas exchange. Additionally, the systemic inflammatory response can escalate muscle wasting and weakness (Barnes & Celli, 2009). Comorbidities such as cardiovascular disease, osteoporosis, metabolic syndrome, depression and anxiety, and diabetes can be exacerbated or worsened due to systemic inflammation (Barnes & Celli, 2009; Muth, 2015).

Asthma effects almost 300 million people worldwide, and about 8% of the U.S. adult population and 10% of the U.S. youth population (Centers for Disease Control and Prevention [CDC], 2011; Lambrecht & Hammad, 2015). Asthma is responsible for 2 million emergency departmnent visits and half a million hospitalizations annually, as well as 9 deaths per day, or almost 3500 deaths annually (CDC, 2011; Muth, 2015). Asthma costs a patient $3300 per year in medical costs, and the total cost (medical and lost productivity) is estimated to be over $18 billion annually (Lambrecht & Hammad, 2015).

Pharmacology and Nutrition

Although quitting smoking is the most effective intervention to alleviate lung function decline associated with COPD, and there is no known cure for asthma, exercise, nutrition, and pharmacology can reduce the burden (Donaire-Gonzalez et al., 2014; Rundell, 2018). Nutrition and drug therapies center around reducing airway inflammation and exercise can reduce bronchial hypertension in asthma patients and help restore activities of daily living for COPD patients. Pharmacological treatments include short and long acting bronchodilators, leukotriene modifiers, and corticosteroids. Table 9.1 lists the various drugs used in the treatment of COPD, side effects, and effects on exercise.

Table 9.1

Pharmacological treatments for asthma and COPD

Type of drug	Type of use	Side effects	Effects of exercise
Short acting B_2AR agonist (SABA)	Acute and chronic Fast acting Lasts 4-6 hours	Headache, tachycardia, tremors, anxiety, nausea, dry mouth, cough	Improves exercise via reduction of symptoms
Long acting B_2AR agonist (LABA)	Maintenance therapy Combination therapy with inhaled corticosteroids	Headache, tachycardia, tremors, anxiety, nausea, dry mouth, cough	Effect unknown due to inconsistent research
Inhaled steroids	Combination therapy with LABAs	Sore throat	n/a
Oral steroids	Short or long term	Fluid retention, hyperglycemia, muscle atrophy, osteoporosis, bruising, myopathy	n/a
Leukotriene modifiers	Alternative for persistent asthma Not recommended for COPD	Headache, cough, irritability Anaphylaxis may occur	Useful in preventing exercise-induced bronchospasm.

Ejiofor & Turner, 2013; Muth, 2015; Rundell et al., 2018

Similar to pharmacotherapy, nutritional considerations should focus on reducing inflammation. Due to the anti-inflammatory properties of some antioxidants, a diet high in fruits and vegetables has been shown to be beneficial for patients who suffer from inflammatory lung diseases (de Boer, van de Worp, Hageman, & Bast, 2017; Muth, 2015). Vitamin E and probiotics may provide the most profound effect on chronic inflammatory lung disease. Other antioxidants that may improve lung function by reducing inflammation are Vitamins A and C. Although there is limited research on Omega-3 and Omega-6 fatty acids, it appears Omega-3 may act as an anti-inflammatory, and Omega-6 may be pro-inflammatory. Additionally, even though there is little effect on inflammation, caffeine is known to improve lung function through bronchodilation.

Activity

The main goal for a client with COPD should be to improve quality of life by reducing barriers to training and activity, and minimize comorbidities (ACSM, 2018; GOLD, 2016; Muth, 2015). However, even though clients with COPD can improve their quality of life, exercise will not cure COPD, and due to the long-lasting nature of the disease, and varying degrees of severity, there is no consensus on FITT principles. Low-moderate intensity exercise can reduce systemic inflammation and increase peripheral vascularity due to the removal of CO_2; increase skeletal muscle function by increasing O_2 levels; and improve self-efficacy. While low-intensity exercise can reduce the risk of future hospital visits, high-intensity exercise may be contraindicated due to an increase in airway inflammatory response (Donaire-Gonzalez et al., 2014; Muth, 2015).

Although exercise reduces systemic inflammation, the effect on airway inflammation in asthma patients is largely unknown. However, because many asthma patients do not exercise at all, any improvement in lung function and strength will be a benefit. Exercise-induced bronchospasms (EIB) occurs when the symptoms of asthma are brought on by exercise or activity. Up to 80% of asthma patients may experience EIB, but it can affect individuals without an underlying diagnosis of asthma and may present symptoms only during exercise (Craig & Dispenza, 2013). In some cases, symptoms may not present until after exercise halts and can last for 12 hours. EIB can be triggered by cold and/or dry air, inhaled or food allergens, pollutants, and a rapid onset of vigorous activity. Consequently, caution should be used during resistance training, and more specifically upper body exercises that increase ventilation such as cross-country skiing, rowing, or hand-cranked ergometers. Conversely, exercise in an indoor and humid environment, such as an indoor pool, may be a good choice. For clients with well controlled asthma, exercise guidelines for the general population can be used.

It is advised a client with COPD who has not participated in a medically-supervised pulmonary rehabilitation program be evaluated for cardiovascular disease risks. Additionally, for clients with COPD or asthma, a medical clearance is recommended, and a 6-minute walk test should be performed as it is easy to complete (Muth, 2015). See the Table 9.2 for FITT guidelines.

The list offers considerations to be used when working with clients with pulmonary dysfunction:

- Only start a bout of exercise if symptoms are under control.
- Perform a 10-15-minute warm-up, and an extended cool down.
- Use RPE scale to communicate severity of symptoms.
- Avoid exercising in areas that contain asthma triggers.
- Incorporate intervals when possible.
- Muscular fatigue may be the most limiting factor for a client with COPD.
- The limitations from dyspnea can be overcome with experience.
- Keep all fast-acting inhalers readily available.
- Optimal time to exercise is late morning.
- Clients should practice pursed-lip and diaphragmatic breathing.

Table 9.2

FITT guidelines for pulmonary dysfunction

FITT for COPD	Frequency	Intensity	Time	Type
Cardiorespiratory	3-5 days/week	Light: 30-40%peak VO2 Vigorous: 60-80% VO2 max Should be based on 6-minute walk test	No less than 15 min Ideally 30-40 min	Walking/cycling
Resistance	2-3 days/week	40-80% 1RM	1-4 sets 8-12 reps	All modalities Mostly large muscle groups

FITT for asthma				
Cardiorespiratory	Start with 2-3 days/ week Progress to 5 days/week	No more than 60% VO2max, or 80% walking speed determined from 6-minute walk test	Start with 20-30 min Progress to 40 minutes	Swimming Walking Running Cycling
Resistance	2-3 days/week	60-80% 1RM	2-4 sets 6-12 reps	All modalities Mostly large muscle groups

ACSM, 2018; Muth, 2015; Rundell, 2018

Discussion and application

1. What is exercise-induced asthma, what is the prevalence, and what are the causes?
2. What is the main goal of exercise therapy for a client with COPD, and what benefits are specific to a client with COPD?

References

American College of Sports Medicine. (2018). *ACSM's resources for the exercise physiologist: A practical guide for the health fitness professional* (P. Magyari, R. Lite, M. W. Kilpatrick, & J. E. Schoffstall Eds. 2 ed.). Philadelphia, PA: Wolters Kluwer.

Barnes, P. J., & Celli, B. R. (2009). Systemic manifestations and comorbidities of *COPD. European Respiratory Journal, 33*(5), 1165-1185. https://doi.org/1010.1183/09031936.00128008

Centers for Disease Control and Prevention. (2011). Asthma in the U.S. Retrieved from https://www.cdc.gov/vitalsigns/asthma/index.html

Craig, T. J., & Dispenza, M. C. (2013). Benefits of exercise in asthma. Annals of Allergy Asthma & Immunology, 110(3), 133-140 e132. https://doi.org/10.1016/j.anai.2012.10.023

de Boer, A., van de Worp, W., Hageman, G. J., & Bast, A. (2017). The effect of dietary components on inflammatory lung diseases—a literature review. *International Journal of Food Sciences and Nutrition, 68*(7), 771-787. https://doi.org/10.1080/09637486.2017.1288199

Donaire-Gonzalez, D., Gimeno-Santos, E., Balcells, E., de Batlle, J., Ramon, M. A., Rodriguez, E.,… Group, P.-C. S. (2015). Benefits of physical activity on COPD hospitalisation depend on intensity. *European Respiratory Journal, 46*(5), 1281-1289. https://doi.org/10.1183/13993003.01699-2014

Ejiofor, S., & Turner, A. M. (2013). Pharmacotherapies for COPD. *Clinical Medicine Insights: Circulatory, Respiratory and Pulmonary Medicine, 7,* 17-34. https://doi.org/10.4137/CCRPM.S7211

Global Initiative for Chronic Obstructive Lung Disease (GOLD). (2016) Global strategy for the diagnosis, management and prevention of COPD. Retrieved from http://goldcopd.org/global-strategy-diagnosis-management-prevention-copd-2016/

Krucik, G. (2018). COPD; Facts, statistics, and you. *Healthline*. Retrieved from https://www.healthline.com/health/copd/facts-statistics-infographic#1

Lambrecht, B. N., & Hammad, H. (2015). The immunology of asthma. *Nature Immunology, 16*(1), 45-56. https://doi.org/10.1038/ni.3049

Muth, N. D. (2015). Pulmonary disease: Asthma and chronic obstructive pulmonary disorder in J.S. Skinner, C.X. Bryant, S. Merrill, & D.J. Green (Eds), *American Council on Exercise medical exercise specialist manual.* San Diego, CA: American Council on Exercise

Rundell, K. W., Smoliga, J. M., & Weiss, P. (2018). Pulmonary disorders and conditions in P.L. Jacobs (Ed) *NSCA's essentials of training special populations*. Champaign, IL: Human Kinetics.

Silkoff, P. E., Strambu, I., Laviolette, M., Singh, D., FitzGerald, J. M., Lam, S.,…Loza, M. J. (2015). Asthma characteristics and biomarkers from the Airways Disease Endotyping for Personalized Therapeutics (ADEPT) longitudinal profiling study. *Respiratory Research, 16*, 142. https://doi.org/10.1186/s12931-015-0299-y

CHAPTER 10
DIABETES

By the end of this chapter you will understand:

- Types of diabetes
  - o Prevalence
  - o Risk factors
- Characteristics and diagnostic criteria
- Treatment strategies
  - o Activity
  - o Pharmacological
  - o Nutrition
- Considerations and contraindications

Background

Diabetes mellitus (DM) affects over 30 million individuals in the United States, and is accountable for almost 80,000 deaths annually, and indirectly accountable for over 250,000 additional deaths. Diabetes is the 7th leading cause of death in the United States with an estimated cost of almost $250 billion annually (Centers for Disease Control and Prevention [CDC], 2017). There are over 1.5 million new cases reported every year, and over 84 million U.S. adults are considered pre-diabetic (CDC, 2017). Risk factors are smoking, obesity or overweight, sedentary lifestyle, high blood pressure, and high cholesterol. Cardiovascular disease, including ischemic heart disease and stroke, is a major complication associated with DM, affecting close to 1.5 million adults. Other complications of DM are lower limb amputation

(100,000+ adults), diabetic ketoacidosis (170,000 adults), abnormal protein metabolism, retinopathy, and neuropathy (CDC, 2017; Verity, 2015)

The incidence of Type I diabetes (T1DM) is only 5-10% of the total of people diagnosed with diabetes, leaving the remaining 90-95% diagnosed with Type II diabetes (T2DM) (Colberg et al., 2016; Verity, 2015). DM results when there is a disruption in the production of insulin, causing hyperglycemia, or increased blood glucose (American College of Sports Medicine [ACSM], 2018). T1DM is an autoimmune disease that damages the pancreas and it does not produce insulin; in T2DM, the pancreas produces insulin, but due to insulin resistance or the lack of sensitivity to insulin in adipose tissue, the liver, or muscle cells, it cannot produce enough, resulting in an absolute or relative lack of insulin.

Diagnostic Criteria

There are a number of tests available to determine a diagnosis of DM. The A1C test measures a person's average blood glucose for the previous 60-90 days, a fasting plasma glucose (FPG) test checks fasting blood glucose levels, an oral glucose tolerance test (OGGT) tests blood glucose levels over a 4-hour period, and a random plasma glucose test checks blood glucose levels at any time of the day. Only a physician can make a diagnosis of diabetes, and testing should take place in a health care facility with professionally trained clinicians. Table 10.1 lists the criteria for a diagnosis of diabetes based on results from the various tests.

Table 10.1

Criteria for diabetes assessments

Method / Result	A1C	FPG	OGTT	Random
Normal	< 5.7	<100mg/dl	<140 mg/dl	n/a
Pre-diabetic	5.7-6.4	100 mg/dl -125 mg/dl	140 mg/dl -199 mg/dl	n/a
Diabetic	≥6.5	≥126 mg/dl	≥200 mg/dl	>200 mg/dl

American Diabetes Association, 2019; Verity, 2015

Treatment Strategies

Exercise

For clients with T1DM, exercise is not an effective means to control blood glucose levels (ACSM, 2018; Verity, 2015). However, because many people with T1DM are often sedentary, overweight or obese, have hypertension or dyslipidemia, it is important for them to maintain a regular exercise schedule. Additionally, because cardiovascular disease is the leading cause of morbidity and mortality in people with T1DM, regular exercise can alleviate or the lower risk of cardio-metabolic disease (Colberg et al., 2016; Riddell et al., 2017; Verity, 2015).

For clients with T1DM, exercise can be used, in addition to proper nutrition and medication, to improve insulin sensitivity and lower A1C. Other benefits include lower blood pressure and cholesterol, weight maintenance or loss, increased energy, improved circulation, and decreased insulin resistance. It is recommended clients with DM be active 5-7 days per week, beginning with 20 minutes per day that can be split into shorter sessions, and progressing to 60 minutes per day, using a combination of aerobic and resistance training (ACSM, 2018). High-intensity interval training (HIIT) can also be used as means to promote skeletal muscle oxidative capacity, insulin sensitivity, and glycemic control for clients with T2DM, and will not hinder glycemic control for clients with T1DM (Colberg et al., 2016). Keep in mind metabolic conditions such as diabetes often occur in conjunction with other chronic conditions such as HTN, CVD, and pulmonary disorders, and the FITT guidelines for comorbid conditions need to be individually considered. FITT Guidelines for clients with diabetes are in Table 10.2.

Table 10.2

FITT guidelines for diabetes

Diabetes	Frequency	Intensity	Time	Type	Notes
Aerobic	3-7 days/week	Moderate to vigorous: 40-80 HRR RPE 12-16	20-60 min/bout 150 min/week moderate 90 min/week vigorous	Exercises that target large muscle groups: Walk, jog, cycle, swim	For clients without contraindications, vigorous intensity, to include HIIT, should be considered
Resistance	2-3 non-consecutive days/week	60-80%1RM RPE 11-15	8-12 exercises 1-4 sets Moderate: 8-12 reps Vigorous: 6-8 Reps	Major muscle groups 4-5 exercises each for upper and lower body	Begin moderately Increase weight and lower reps, then increase sets, and then the number of bouts
Flexibility	2-3 days/week	Stretch to ROM tightness	15-30 sec/stretch 2-4 reps/stretch	4-5 exercises each for upper and lower body	Can perform static or dynamic and increase time or reps as is warranted by progress
Neuromuscular	2-3 days/week	Light to moderate	Incorporate into other workouts	Single leg functional movements Yoga, Tai Chi	Increase time or reps as progress is warranted

ASCM, 2018; Colberg et al., 2016; LaFontaine, Roitman, & Sorace, 2018; Verity, 2015

Exercise and Medications

There are several medications prescribed for diabetes that control symptoms (Table 10.3). For example, hypoglycemia is a common occurrence for diabetics; particularly during exercise. Clients with T1DM do not have a uniform response to exercise; therefore, determining a dose-response relationship to exercise is difficult, and exercise may prompt a hypoglycemic event. While aerobic exercise is known to decrease blood glucose levels, resistance training is known to lessen the risk of exercise-induced hypoglycemia. To reduce the chance of exercise-induced hypoglycemia for clients with T1DM, resistance exercise is recommended prior to aerobic exercise (Colberg et al., 2016). For clients with T2DM, exercise can result in lower blood glucose levels, and the more physical activity that is performed, the lower the insulin resistance and the greater the insulin sensitivity. Additionally, clients with T2DM can suffer from abnormal insulin secretion, and when coupled with exercise, may result in hyperinsulinemia instigating a hypoglycemic event. Continuous glucose monitoring can determine a hypoglycemic event, allowing appropriate action if needed.

Table 10.3

Common diabetes medications

Medication	Mechanics	Side effects	Exercise considerations
Type I diabetes			
Insulin Sort, intermediate, and fast acting	Supplies insulin because the pancreas is does not	Injection site irritation Hypoglycemia	Injected insulin may release faster during exercise Exercise increase glucose uptake which may result in hypoglycemia
Pramlintide	Blunts blood glucose levels following eating	Injection site irritation Poor appetite Lethargy	May result in decreased performance
Type II diabetes			
Insulin	Supplies insulin when the pancreas is unable to	Injection site irritation Hypoglycemia	Injected insulin may release faster during exercise Exercise increase glucose uptake which may result in hypoglycemia
Sulfonylureas	Stimulates pancreas to release insulin	Hypoglycemia Weight gain Nausea	Risk of hypoglycemia Blood sugar levels need to be monitored during first few sessions, until response to exercise can be predicted
DPP4 inhibitors	Stimulates the release of insulin Inhibits the release of glucose from the liver	Respiratory tract infection Headache	Unknown Possibly hypoglycemia
Biguanide	Improves insulin sensitivity Inhibits the release of glucose from the liver	Nausea Diarrhea	Exercise may hinder drug actions May increase heart rate response to exercise
Thiazolidinedione	Improves insulin sensitivity Inhibits the release of glucose from the liver	Cardiac events Liver disease	Strong possibility of hypoglycemia
Alpha-glucose inhibitors	Slows the breakdown and absorption of carbohydrates	GI distress Diarrhea	Strong possibility of hypoglycemia

LaFontaine et al., 2018

Dietary Considerations

Lifestyle in intervention is critical to mitigate the consequences of DM, as well as prevent, delay, or reverse comorbidities. For clients with prediabetes a reduction of 5-7% of bodyweight is suggested combined with the recommended exercise (Table 10.2) can delay the progression to T2DM by almost 60% (Dyson et al., 2011; Verity, 2015). A CXS needs to be aware of any dietary restrictions or modifications as these may have an effect on exercise performance. The following guidelines summarize recommendations for the prevention of prediabetes and the management of DM (Asif, 2014; Dyson et al., 2011; LaFontaine et al., 2018. Verity, 2015).

Everyone with prediabetes or diabetes should consult a registered dietician.

- Weight loss should be the main goal
    - o Energy restriction
    - o Low-fat diets
    - o Increased physical activity
    - o Monitor glucose and carbohydrate consumption and adjust insulin accordingly
- Diets should be low glycemic and high in fiber
- Vegan diets can moderate the effects of diabetes by up to 43%
- Diets should include
    - o Low-fat dairy foods
    - o Green leafy vegetables
    - o Carbohydrates should be starch (rice, beans, potatoes)
    - o Moderate alcohol consumption
- Foods to avoid are
    - o Red meats
    - o Animal fats
    - o Processed products
    - o Refined sugar except during sever hypoglycemic episodes
    - o Fried foods
    - o Salt
- Micronutrient considerations
    - o Plant sterols and stanols may benefit blood lipid profile
    - o Vitamins A, C, E, or carotene may be harmful
    - o Limit sodium to 2300mg/day

Complications and Concerns

Microvascular or neural disease are common complications of diabetes, and even though regular exercise may prevent or delay onset, it is prudent to be aware of neuropathy, retinopathy, and nephropathy. Neuropathy is weakness, numbness, and pain from nerve damage, usually in the hands or feet. If a client has been diagnosed with neuropathy, to mitigate skeletomuscular injuries, particularly in the extremities, avoiding vigorous exercise such as plyometrics is advised. Accordingly, incorporating non-weight bearing exercise may be prudent. Cardiac autonomic neuropathy can exacerbate cardiovascular disorders in diabetics, including a blunted heart rate response, and sudden variations in orthostatic blood pressure. Using the RPE scale to determine intensity may be necessary, and sudden postural or directional changes should be avoided (Colberg et al., 2016). Clients with DM have a high risk for retinopathy, or retinal detachment. Clients diagnosed with retinopathy should avoid high intensity exercise and limit systolic blood pressure to 20-30 mmHg above resting. Nephropathy, or kidney damage, is experienced by 30% of diabetics, and the risk is increased as blood pressure rises. Clients with nephropathy can benefit from low intensity exercise and should limit SBP to 180-200 mmHg. High-intensity weight training that may induce the Valsalva maneuver should be avoided (Verity, 2015). For most clients with DM, the benefits of exercise outweigh the involved risks, but a CXS should be aware of the precautions listed below:

- Be cautious of the side effects of medication.
- Hypoglycemia may occur as a response to exercise in clients with T2DM as a result of hyperinsulinemia
- Previously sedentary clients may need to start at a very low intensity for both aerobic and resistance training.
- It may be necessary to use RPE for clients with diabetes because of an altered max HR due to cardiac autonomic neuropathy.
- A medical clearance is not always necessary for asymptomatic clients, but due to the risk of a cardiac event, it is prudent to get clearance.
- A medically supervised exercise test may need to be performed prior to beginning an exercise program—consult with a client's physician.
- Hypoglycemia is the most common response to exercise (a blood glucose of >70 mg/dl). Symptoms include profuse sweating, cold and clammy skin and appearance, persistent shaking, confusion, slurred speech, and dizziness or fainting.
- If a client is displaying hypoglycemic symptoms, a simple sugar snack containing 20-30 grams of carbohydrates can help.
- For a client with diabetes, 15-30 grams of carbohydrates should be consumed every 30 minutes of moderate exercise.
- Blood glucose should be monitored prior to, during, and after exercise.
- Be cautious of dehydration.
- Clients with retinopathy or neuropathy should avoid vigorous exercise due to a higher risk for retinal detachment and hemorrhage.

- Because 75% of individuals with T2DM will die from a cardiovascular event, be cautious and aware when performing vigorous exercise

Discussion and application

1. Identify the components of a medical team, and how a Health and Fitness Professional fits into the overall medical team to address a client/patient with diabetes.
2. Define and discuss ways to avoid exercise-induced hyperglycemia and post-exercise hypoglycemia.

References

American College of Sports Medicine. (2018). *ACSM's resources for the exercise physiologist: A practical guide for the health fitness professional* (P. Magyari, R. Lite, M. W. Kilpatrick, & J. E. Schoffstall Eds. 2 ed.). Philadelphia, PA: Wolters Kluwer.

American Diabetes Association. (2019). Diagnosing diabetes and learning about prediabetes. Retrieved from http://www.diabetes.org/diabetes-basics/diagnosis/

Asif, M. (2014). The prevention and control the type-2 diabetes by changing lifestyle and dietary pattern. *Journal of Education and Health Promotion, 3*, 1. https://doi.org/10.4103/2277-9531.127541

Centers for Disease Control and Prevention. (2017). *National diabetes statistics report, 2017*. Atlanta, GA: Centers for Disease Control and Prevention and U.S. Department of Health and Human Services.

Colberg, S. R., Sigal, R. J., Yardley, J. E., Riddell, M. C., Dunstan, D. W., Dempsey, P. C.,...Tate, D. F. (2016). Physical activity/exercise and diabetes: A position statement of the American diabetes association. *Diabetes Care, 39*(11), 2065-2079. https://doi.org/10.2337/dc16-1728

Dyson, P. A., Kelly, T., Deakin, T., Duncan, A., Frost, G., Harrison, Z.,...Diabetes, U. K. N. W. G. (2011). Diabetes UK evidence-based nutrition guidelines for the prevention and management of diabetes. *Diabetic Medicine, 28*(11), 1282-1288. https://doi.org/10.1111/j.1464-5491.2011.03371.x

LaFontaine, L., Roitman, J. l, & Sorace, P. (2018). Metabolic conditions and disorders in P.L. Jacobs (Ed) *NSCA's essentials of training special populations*. Champaign, IL: Human Kinetics.

Riddell, M. C., Gallen, I. W., Smart, C. E., Taplin, C. E., Adolfsson, P., Lumb, A. N.,...Laffel, L. M. (2017). Exercise management in type 1 diabetes: A consensus statement. *The Lancet Diabetes & Endocrinology, 5*(5), 377-390. https://doi.org/10.1016/s2213-8587(17)30014-1

Verity, L. S. (2015). Diabetes mellitus in J.S. Skinner, C.X. Bryant, S. Merrill, & D.J. Green (Eds), *American Council on Exercise medical exercise specialist manual*. San Diego, CA: American Council on Exercise.

CHAPTER 11
HYPERLIPIDEMIA

By the end of this chapter you will understand:

- Cholesterol and triglycerides
- Recommended goals for blood lipids
- Treatments:
    - o Exercise
    - o Nutrition
    - o Pharmacological
- FITT guidelines for blood lipid disorders

Cholesterol and Triglycerides

Hyperlipidemia, or *dyslipidemia* is a term to describe abnormal blood fat and lipoproteins (American College of Sports Medicine [ACSM], 2018; LaFontaine, Roitman, & Sorace, 2018). Lipoproteins are protein and fats that bind together and travel through the blood, carrying cholesterol (a waxy fat) and triglycerides. Triglycerides are made of three molecules of fatty acid and a molecule of glycerin, and are the most common fat in the body. In normal amounts cholesterol is a source of energy for the body, and triglycerides, in addition to being a fuel source help build cells (Mayo Clinic, 2019; Sugerman, 2013). However, at elevated levels, cholesterol builds in artery walls and disrupts normal blood flow, while triglycerides are associated with elevated cholesterol, and cardiovascular disease (CVD) risk factors such as obesity and metabolic syndrome. In combination, elevated levels of cholesterol and triglycerides are risk factors for atherosclerotic cardiovascular disease (ASCVD), a comprehensive term to describe multiple cardiovascular events caused by atherosclerosis including coronary heart disease (CHD), angina, stroke, and myocardial infarctions (Ference et al., 2017; La Forge, 2015). Comorbidities associated with dyslipidemia are:

- Chronic heart disease
- Angina
- Diabetes
- Hypertension
- Obesity
- Metabolic syndrome
- Insulin resistance
- Renal Disease
- Peripheral vascular disease
- Chronic obstructive pulmonary disease

There are a number of classes of plasma lipoproteins, based on size and lipid composition, however, we will only discuss the five in Table 11.1.

Table 11.1

Classes and composition of plasma lipoproteins

Lipoprotein	Density (g/ml)	Size (nm)	Major Lipids	Composition
Chylomicrons	<0.930	75-1200	Triglycerides	Large triglyceride rich particles made by the intestine. They transport dietary triglycerides and cholesterol from the intestines to peripheral tissues and the liver.
Very low-density lipoproteins (VLDL)	0.930-1.006	30-80	Triglycerides Serum Cholesterol	Produced by the liver and are triglyceride rich and carry up to 15% of the body's serum cholesterol.
Intermediate-density lipoprotein (IDL)	1.006-1.019	25-35	Triglycerides Cholesterol	Remnants formed when triglycerides are deposited in muscle cells and adipose tissue by VLDL. IDLs also contain significant amounts of cholesterol, and along with VLDL, contribute to ASCVD.
Low-density lipoproteins (LDL)	1.019-1.063	18-25	Cholesterol	Carry approximately 60-70% of blood cholesterol and are formed from the catabolism of VLDLs. Due to the contribution to atherosclerosis, LDLs are considered the bad cholesterol.
High-density lipoproteins (HDL)	1.063-1.210	5-12	Cholesterol Phospholipids	Carry cholesterol from the blood back to the liver. Because of this reverse transport process, HDLs are consider the good or healthy cholesterol.

Feingold & Grunfeld, 2018; LaFontaine et al., 2018; La Forge, 2015

Recently, rather than using LDL cholesterol as a marker for CVD, non-HDL cholesterol levels and total cholesterol to HDL ratios have been studied. Because non-HDL cholesterol levels include other potentially harmful lipoproteins, it is considered a more comprehensive measurement when considering CVD risk factors. Similarly, total cholesterol to HDL ratios may also be a more valid predictor of CVD than just total cholesterol as it considers the benefits of a higher HDL level (Lopez-Jimenez, 2019). Accordingly, higher ratios mean a higher risk of heart disease. Ideally, the ratio should be below 5.0, with the optimum ratio at 3.5 (Mosca, 2007). However, while the total cholesterol to HDL ratio can be used as a guideline, it is not generally used for treatment. Table 11.2 details lipid level guidelines.

Table 11.2

Lipid level guidelines

Lipid in mg/dl	Optimal	Near optimal	Borderline	High	Very High
Total Cholesterol	<150	<200	200-239	>240	
LDL	<100	100-129	130-159	160-189	>190
HDL	>60			<40	
Triglycerides	<100	<150	150-199	200-499	>500

ACSM, 2019; Harvard Medical School, 2015; La Fontaine et al., 2018

Exercise

Regardless of the dangers of high levels of lipoproteins, lipids are a primary source of energy for aerobic and endurance exercise, and a modest source of energy for resistance exercise. Fatty acids are mobilized from adipose tissue and transported to working muscles. Different forms of exercise will result in reductions in total cholesterol, triglycerides, and LDL cholesterol, and an increase in HDL cholesterol. Triglycerides are particularly responsive to exercise, and mostly decrease immediately after exercise. Consequently, moderate to vigorous exercise 1-12 hours prior to a meal rich in fats can lower postprandial triglycerides (Gordon, Chen, & Durstine, 2014; La Forge, 2015). Long-term resistance exercise programs (>12 weeks) can result in up to a 3% decrease in total cholesterol, a 4.5% decrease in LDL, a 6% decrease in non-HDL cholesterol, and a 6% decrease in triglycerides. Resistance training can increase HDL cholesterol by approximately 1%. Because aerobic exercise uses lipids as a primary energy source, it can lead to a decrease of 2% in total cholesterol, 2.5% in non-HDL cholesterol, and 11% in triglycerides. Aerobic exercise can also lead to a 4% increase in HDL cholesterol (Gordon et al., 2014). Exercise recommendations for clients suffering from blood lipid disorders are detailed in Table 11.3.

Table 11.3

FITT guidelines for clients with blood lipid disorders

Mode	Frequency	Intensity	Time	Type
Aerobic	5-7 days/week	40-75 HRR RPE 12-16	15-60 min/bout Can be performed in 10 min. bouts With a long-term goal of at least 300 min/week and a total caloric expenditure goal of 2000cal./week	Exercises that target large muscle groups: Walk, jog, cycle, swim
Resistance	2-3 non-consecutive days/week	60-80%1RM RPE 11-15	8-12 exercises 8-12 reps 1-4 sets	Major muscle groups 4-5 exercises each for upper and lower body
Flexibility	3-7 days/week	Stretch to ROM tightness	10-30 sec/stretch 2-3 reps/stretch	4-5 exercises each for upper and lower body

ACSM; 2018; LaFontaine, 2018; La Forge, 2015

Nutrition

Although this manual is not intended to replace an educated and experienced nutritionist or registered dietician, proper nutrition habits combined with exercise, and in many cases pharmacological therapy, help with the management of dyslipidemia. There are a number of diets that provide guidance including eating plans developed by the American Heart Association and also by the Office of Disease Prevention and Health Promotion (LaFontaine, 2018; La Forge, 2015; Lichtenstein, et al., 2006; U.S. Department of Health and Human Services, 2019). General guidelines are:

- Lose body fat if needed (8-10 pounds can reduce LDL by up to 8%).
- Consume no more than 7% of calories from saturated fat (can reduce LDL by up to 10%).
- Avoid trans-fat.
- Only consume 20-30% of calories from fat sources.
- Consume no more than 200mg of cholesterol daily (can reduce LDL by up to 5%).
- Consume 25gm of berries daily.
- Consume fish for 2-3 meals per week.
- Consume 25gm of soy protein daily.
- Consume 5-10 gm of soluble fiber daily (can reduce LDL by up to 5%).
- Limit sugars to less than 5% of daily calories.
- Limit processed foods.

- Limit alcohol to 2 or fewer drinks per day.
- Consume 2gm of plant stanols and sterols daily (can reduce LDL by up to 15%).

Medication

Clients with blood lipid disorders may be prescribed medication by a physician. Some medications have undesirable side effects and some may interfere with the benefits of exercise. Table 11.4 lists common medications, their purpose, and side effects.

Table 11.4

Common medications for dyslipidemia and their side effects

Drug Class	Purpose	Side Effects	Effects on Exercise
HMG-CoA reductase inhibitors (AKA Statins)	Disrupt cholesterol synthesis to lower LDL	GI issues, headaches, muscle aches, dizziness, myopathy	May reduce the effectiveness of aerobic exercise May increase myalgia (muscle pain and/or damage) with exercise
Niacin	Lowers LDL and triglycerides, but most beneficial for increasing HDL	Flushing, itching, hypotension	No known effects
Fibrates	Lower triglycerides and increase HDL	GI issues, muscle aches, rash	May increase myalgia (muscle pain and/or damage) with exercise
Bile acid sequestrants	Bind bile acids to lower total and LDL cholesterol	GI issues	No known effects
Cholesterol absorption blockers	Blocks cholesterol from being absorbed and lowers total plasma cholesterol	GI issues	No known effects
Omega-3	Lowers triglycerides	No known side effects	No known effects

La Forge, 2015; LaFontaine et al., 2018

Discussion and application

1. Define the types of lipoproteins. Discuss each role as well as the benefits or disadvantages.
2. Explain the benefits of exercise on cholesterol levels.

References

American College of Sports Medicine. (2018). *ACSM's resources for the exercise physiologist: A practical guide for the health fitness professional* (P. Magyari, R. Lite, M. W. Kilpatrick, & J. E. Schoffstall Eds. 2 ed.). Philadelphia, PA: Wolters Kluwer.

Feingold, K. R., & Grunfeld, C. (2018). Introduction to lipids and lipoproteins. In K. R. Feingold, B. Anawalt, A. Boyce, & et al (Eds.), *Endotext [Internet].* South Dartmouth, MA: MDText.com, Inc.

Ference, B. A., Ginsberg, H. N., Graham, I., Ray, K. K., Packard, C. J., Bruckert, E.,…Catapano, A. L. (2017). Low-density lipoproteins cause atherosclerotic cardiovascular disease. 1. Evidence from genetic, epidemiologic, and clinical studies. A consensus statement from the European Atherosclerosis Society Consensus Panel. *European Heart Journal, 38*(32), 2459-2472. https://doi.org/10.1093/eurheartj/ehx144

Gordon, B., Chen, S., & Durstine, J. L. (2014). The effects of exercise training on the traditional lipid profile and beyond. *Current Sports Medicine Reports, 13*(4), 253-259. https://doi.org/10.1249/JSR.0000000000000073

Harvard Medical School. (2015). Making sense of cholesterol tests: The pros and cons of total cholesterol, HDL, LDL, and triglyceride testing. Retrieved from https://www.health.harvard.edu/heart-health/making-sense-of-cholesterol-tests

LaFontaine, L., Roitman, J. l, & Sorace, P. (2018). Metabolic conditions and disorders in P.L. Jacobs (Ed) *NSCA's essentials of training special populations.* Champaign, IL: Human Kinetics.

LaForge, R. (2015). Blood lipid disorders in J.S. Skinner, C.X. Bryant, S. Merrill, & D.J. Green (Eds), *American Council on Exercise medical exercise specialist manual.* San Diego, CA: American Council on Exercise.

Lichtenstein, A. H., Appel, L. J., Brands, M., Carnethon, M., Daniels, S., Franch, H. A.,…& Karanja, N. (2006). Diet and lifestyle recommendations revision 2006: a scientific statement from the American Heart Association Nutrition Committee. *Circulation, 114*(1), 82-96. https://doi.org/10.1161/CIRCULATIONAHA.106.176158

Lopez-Jimenez, F. (2019). Cholesterol ratio or non-HDL cholesterol: Which is most important. Retrieved from https://www.mayoclinic.org/diseases-conditions/high-blood-cholesterol/expert-answers/cholesterol-ratio/faq-20058006

Mayo Clinic. (2019). Triglycerides: Why do they matter. Retrieved from https://www.mayoclinic.org/diseases-conditions/high-blood-cholesterol/in-depth/triglycerides/art-20048186

Mosca, L. (2007). Total cholesterol to HDL ratio. *Everyday Health.* Retrieved from https://www.everydayhealth.com/specialists/cardio/mosca/total-cholesterol-to-hdl-ratio/index.aspx

Sugerman, D. T. (2013). Blood lipids: JAMA patient page. *JAMA, 310*(16), 1751-1751. https://doi.org/10.1001/jama.2013.280593

U.S. Department of Health and Human Services. (2019). *Dietary guidelines 2015-2020: Developing the dietary guidelines for Americans.* Retrieved from https://health.gov/dietaryguidelines/2015/guidelines/introduction/developing-the-dietary-guidelines-for-americans/

CHAPTER 12
BODY COMPOSITION, OVERWEIGHT AND OBESITY

By the end of this chapter you will understand:

- Statistics
- Comorbidities
- Body composition measurements
    - o Percentage
    - o BMI
    - o Waist measurements
    - o Hip to waist ratio
- Thermal activity and metabolism
- Treatment strategies
    - o Nutrition
    - o Pharmacological and surgery
    - o Activity
- Risks and contraindications
- FITT

Statistics

Obesity is a growing concern for the United States; to such an extent, it is now considered a chronic disease of its own. The adult obesity rate in the United States is now close to 40% and effects over 93 million Americans (Hales, Carroll, Fryar, & Ogden, 2017). The youth obesity rate is over 18%; up almost 5% in just 10 years. The annual medical cost and lost productivity from obesity is estimated to be over $1.7 trillion. This equates to an estimated per capita cost of over $1400 per year more than adults of normal weight (Centers for Disease Control and Prevention, 2017; Waters & Graf, 2018). Obesity can lead to cardiovascular disease (CVD) such as coronary heart disease (CHD), and stroke, metabolic conditions such as systemic inflammation, diabetes, and dyslipidemia, and pulmonary conditions such as emphysema, and some cancers (Jensen et al, 2014).

Body Composition Metrics

In addition to adipose tissue, body fat is found in almost all tissue including nerves, bone marrow, and organs. This body fat is considered essential for physiological functions. The remainder of fat is stored and used as the primary source of energy. When there is a positive energy balance (caloric intake is greater than caloric expenditure), accumulating fat leads to harmful excess adipose tissue, and ultimately an individual will become overweight and then obese. Essential body fat is around 3% for men, and 12% for women. Other body fat classifications are in Table 12.1.

Table 12.1

Body fat classifications

Males	Females	Rating
3	12	Essential
5-10	8-15	Athletic
11-14	16-23	Good
15-20	24-30	Acceptable
21-24	31-36	Overweight
>24	>37	Obese

(Jensen et al., 2014; Jeukendrup & Gleeson, 2019; Kravitz, 2015).

There are a number of metrics to determine if an individual is overweight or obese. Body mass index, or BMI, is a common tool based on height to weight. BMI = Weight (kg)/Height^2 (m) or [Weight (lb.)/ Height^2 (in)] x 703. BMI should only be used as a guide and not for diagnostic purposes as it cannot distinguish fat mass from fat-free mass. There are charts available for download, as well as online calculators to calculate BMI. It is important to know a BMI of greater than 30 (obese) is considered a risk factor for CVD. The list details BMI categories (American College of Sports Medicine [ACSM], 2018; Jensen et al., 2014; Kravitz, 2015):

Weight	**BMI**	**Weight**	**BMI**
Underweight	<18.5	Obese	30-34.9
Normal Weight	18.5-24.9	Grade II Obesity	35-39.9
Overweight	25-29.9	Grade III Obesity	>40

Recently, attention has been given to central obesity, or visceral fat, found in the abdominal cavity. Because of its location near vital organs, excess visceral fat can contribute to health conditions such as hormonal imbalances, CVD, and metabolic diseases. Accordingly, because visceral fat is located in the abdominal cavity, waist circumference is used as a marker of metabolic health risk (Smith, 2015), and is an adjunct to BMI. For overweight and obese individuals (a BMI of > 25), waist measurements can provide insight to increased health risk (Fahey, Insel, & Roth, 2015; Jensen et al., 2014; Kravitz, 2015). Conversely, because BMI cannot differentiate between fat mass and fat-free mass, it may overestimate body fat in individuals with a muscular build. Therefore, if an individual has a BMI higher than expected, a small waist circumference may indicate a lower health risk due to a higher amount of fat-free mass. It should be noted a waist circumference of greater than 40" for males, and 35" for females is considered a separate risk factor for CVD. The waist circumference and the level of risk are listed in Table 12.2.

Table 12.2

Waist circumference and level of risk

	Normal	Increased risk	Substantial Risk
Men	>37in	37-40in	>40in
Women	>32in	32-35in	>35in

Fahey et al., 2015; Jensen et al., 2014; Kravitz, 2015

In addition to waist circumference, waist to hip ratio has also been found to be a better indicator of CVD and metabolic health risk than BMI alone as it is more indicative of intra-abdominal fat. Increased intra-abdominal fat has been determined to be a marker for increased ectopic fat, or fat formed by triglycerides, and stored in the liver, muscle cells, heart, and pancreas. Ectopic fat can disrupt normal metabolic processes and mitochondrial function, and is associated with insulin resistance that disrupts normal organ function (Smith, 2015). Hip to waist ratio norms for men and women are listed in Tables 12.3 and 12.4.

Table 12.3

Hip to waist ratio norms for men

Age	Low risk	Moderate risk	High risk
20-29	<0.83	0.83-0.88	>0.88
30-39	<0.84	0.84-0.91	>0.91
40-49	<0.88	0.88-0.95	>0.95
50-59	<0.90	0.90-.098	>0.96
60+	<0.91	0.91-0.98	>0.98

ACSM, 2018; Graham & Whitehead, 2018

Table 12.4

Hip to waist ratio norms for women

Age	Low risk	Moderate risk	High risk
20-29	<0.71	0.71-0.77	>0.77
30-39	<0.72	0.72-0.78	>0.78
40-49	<0.73	0.73-0.79	>0.79
50-59	<0.74	0.74-0.81	>0.81
60+	<0.76	0.76-0.83	>0.83

ACSM, 2018; Graham & Whitehead, 2018

Thermal Activity and Metabolism

When discussing caloric expenditure, it is important to understand how the body burns energy and the involvement of each component. Total energy expenditure (TEE) is the total energy expended, and can be divided into four categories: the thermal effect of metabolism (TEM), the thermal effect of food (TEF), the thermal effect of activity (TEA), and non-exercise activity thermogenesis (NEAT) (Trexler, Smith-Ryan, & Norton, 2014). TEM is based on an individual's basal metabolic rate, the bodily functions necessary for life, and accounts for 60–70% of TEE. TEF is the energy required to consume and digest food, and accounts for about 10% of TEE. TEA is the energy associated with activity and accounts for 20-30% of TEE. NEAT is activities such as fidgeting, standing, and walking and can account for half of TEA. Because TEM and TEF are generally consistent, controllable caloric expenditure is predominantly through TEA and NEAT (Trexler, et al., 2014; Villablanca et al., 2015).

Resting metabolic rate (RMR) and fat free mass (FFM) are interconnected, as skeletal muscle comprises of almost 51% of FFM, and contributes 18–25% of RMR (Alexander, 2002; St-Onge & Gallagher, 2010). It should also be noted with aging men may have up to a 5% reduction in RMR per decade, and a reduction in TEA of up to 7.5%. Similarly, women may have up to a 3% reduction in RMR per decade, and a reduction of up to 6% of TEA (St-Onge & Gallagher, 2010). The importance of this cannot be overstated and underscores the importance of a healthy amount of FFM.

Weight Loss and Dietary Guidelines

According to the ACSM (2018), the primary contributing factors to obesity are increased caloric intake and decreased caloric expenditure or physical activity. Accordingly, lifestyle modifications including dietary adjustments, regular exercise, and behavior therapy are all used to reduce and treat the obesity (Burke & Wang, 2011). Behavior change should include strategies such as goal setting, self-monitoring, stimulus control, and cognitive restructuring. Additionally, for consistent weight loss, adherences to a healthy eating plan is more important than the type of diet (Burke & Wang, 2011). A pound is about 3500 calories. Accordingly, to lose one pound per week, a deficit of 500 calories per day needs to be achieved. Keep in mind the 3500-calorie figure is a starting place as caloric expenditure occurs in a non-linear fashion based on individual thermogenics, and actual caloric expenditure may be more or less. Regardless, safe weight loss is no more than 2 pounds, roughly 7000 calories per week or 1000cal/day. General guidelines include (Burke & Wang, 2011; Kravits, 2015; Phelan & Wing, 2005):

- Eat breakfast daily.

- Adhere to consistent eating patterns and times.
- Limit calories to no more than 1500/day for women and 1800/day for men.
- Limit fat to 25-35% of daily calories.
    - o Less than 7% from saturated fat.
    - o Less than 1% from trans-fat.
- Consume fruits and vegetables.
- Consume whole grains.
- Choose high fiber foods.
- Choose lean meat.
- Choose vegetable sources of protein.
- Reduce/minimize food and beverages with added sugar.
- Choose foods with little or no added salt.

Pharmacology and Surgery

There are a number of drugs to aid in weight loss for morbidly obese individuals (Kravitz, 2015). The main function of these drugs is to block the intestines from absorbing dietary fats. Even though there has been some success with mild weight loss, a reduction of blood pressure, and lowering LDL cholesterol, other side effects can be difficult to manage. The most evident side effect is gastrointestinal distress ranging from mild gas, to abdominal pain, to severe diarrhea. Until there is a drug to induce weight loss effectively and safely, a combination of a healthy diet, a consistent exercise program, and behavior change will most likely provide the best results.

Bariatric surgery has become synonymous with bypass surgery, and can include gastric bypass, sleeve gastrectomy or envelope, banding, or an intragastric balloon. Some individuals undergoing bariatric surgery require an invasive procedure, and other individuals have outpatient procedures with little to no down time. Currently, it is not clear, other than recovery time, if a different exercise prescription should be administered to bariatric patients (ACSM, 2018). For clients who have undergone surgery, consulting with a physician and a registered dietician is strongly recommended.

Exercise

The main goal of an exercise program for an obese client is to achieve and maintain a negative energy balance, and the most effective means to accomplish this is via cardiovascular exercise. Although resistance training has numerous health benefits including a reduction of systemic inflammation, and when performed in conjunction with aerobic exercise can increase lean muscle and FFM, the primary focus of a training program for an obese client should be aerobic exercise. Furthermore, rather than counting steps or calories, a gradual increase of up to 60 minutes per day in exercise appears to provide the caloric expenditure necessary for weight loss and to prevent the relapse (ACSM, 2018, Kravitz, 2015). As with most chronic conditions, there are considerations when working with an obese client.

- Non-weight bearing exercise such as a bicycle or swimming may be a more effective place to start than weight bearing exercise such as walking or an elliptical.
- Many clients will need to start slow and gradually progress.
- Low-impact exercise are necessary to avoid musculoskeletal injuries.
- If needed, start with as few as 10 minutes per day and progress to 60 minutes per day.
- Biomechanics may be altered.
    - o To avoid joint stress, an increase in duration of exercise is preferred to an increase of intensity.
    - o Clients may need demonstrations and modifications of exercises.
- Muscular strength and endurance should be used as an adjunct to aerobic conditioning.
- Protocols for each comorbidity need to be recognized and implemented as needed.

FITT recommendations for overweight and obese clients are listed in Table 12.5.

Table 12.5

FITT recommendations for overweight and obese

	Frequency	Intensity	Time	Type
Aerobic	≥ 5 days/week to maximize caloric expenditure	40-60% HRR with the goal of reaching ≥ 60% HRR RPE 12-13	30 min/day with a goal of reaching 60 min/day Limited capacity: 3-6 10-min bouts/day to accumulate 30-60 min/day	Rhythmic activities that target large muscle groups: Walking Cycling Swimming
Resistance Start with recommendations for a healthy, yet deconditioned adult, and progress accordingly	Each major muscle group 2-3 days/week	Light intensity; 40-50% 1RM	10–15 reps for strength 15-20 reps for muscular endurance A single set can be effective	Resistance exercises involving each major muscle group, targeting larger groups first

Flexibility	≥ 2-3 days/week	Stretch to the point of feeling tightness or slight discomfort	Static stretching hold for 10-30 sec. or up to 60 sec. for older individuals For PNF stretching, a 3- to 6-sec contraction at 20%–75% maximum voluntary contraction followed by a 10-30 sec. assisted stretch	Static flexibility, Dynamic flexibility PNF
Neuromuscular exercise training The effectiveness of neuromuscular exercise training in younger and middle-aged persons has not been Established	≥2-3 days/week	N/A	≥20-30 min/bout	Exercise that challenges motor skills, coordination, and proprioception such as Yoga or Tai Chi

ACSM, 2018, Garber, 2011; Graham & Whitehead, 2018; Kravitz, 2015

Discussion and application

1. How do you, in plain words, using evidence-based research explain to a new client why lean muscle is so important in weight loss?
2. What are some concerns that need to be addressed when designing an exercise program for an obese client?

References

Alexander, J. L. (2002). The role of resistance exercise in weight loss. *Strength & Conditioning Journal, 24*(1), 65-69. Retrieved from https://journals.lww.com/nsca-scj/toc/2002/02000

American College of Sports Medicine. (2018). *ACSM's resources for the exercise physiologist: A practical guide for the health fitness professional* (P. Magyari, R. Lite, M. W. Kilpatrick, & J. E. Schoffstall Eds. 2 ed.). Philadelphia, PA: Wolters Kluwer.

Burke, L. E., & Wang, J. (2011). Treatment strategies for overweight and obesity. *Journal of Nursing Scholarship, 43*(4), 368-375. https://doi.org/10.1111/j.1547-5069.2011.01424.x

Centers for Disease Control and Prevention. (2017). Overweight and obesity: Adult obesity facts. Retrieved from https://www.cdc.gov/obesity/data/adult.html

Fahey, T. D., Insel, P. M., & Roth, W. T. (2015). *Fit & well: Core concepts and labs in physical fitness and wellness* (11 ed.). New York, NY: McGraw-Hill Education.

Graham, J. F. & Whitehead, M. T. (2018). Health appraisal and fitness assessments in P.L. Jacobs (Ed*)* *NSCA's essentials of training special populations*. Champaign, IL: Human Kinetics.

Garber, C. E., Blissmer, B., Deschenes, M. R., Franklin, B. A., Lamonte, M. J., Lee, I. M.,...Swain, D. P. (2011). Quantity and quality of exercise for developing and maintaining cardiorespiratory, musculoskeletal, and neuromotor fitness in apparently healthy adults: Guidance for prescribing exercise. *Medical Science in Sports and Exercise, 43*(7), 1334-1359. https://doi.org/10.1249/MSS.0b013e318213fefb

Hales, C. M., Carroll, M. D., Fryar, C. D., & Ogden, C. L. (2017). *NCHS data brief: Prevalence of obesity among adults and youth: United States, 2015–2016 (288)*. Hyattsville, MD: National Center for Health Statistics.

Jensen, M. D., Ryan, D. H., Apovian, C. M., Ard, J. D., Comuzzie, A. G., Donato, K. A.,...Yanovski, S. Z. (2014). 2013 AHA/ACC/TOS Guideline for the Management of Overweight and Obesity in Adults. *Circulation, 129*(25 suppl 2), S102-S138. https://doi.org/10.1161/01.cir.0000437739.71477.ee

Jeukendrup, A., & Gleeson, M. (2019). Normal ranges of body weight and body fat. *In sport nutrition* (pp. 415-416). Champaign, IL: Human Kinetics.

Kravitz, L. (2015). Overweight and obesity in J.S. Skinner, C.X. Bryant, S. Merrill, & D.J. Green (Eds), *American Council on Exercise medical exercise specialist manual*. San Diego, CA: American Council on Exercise.

La Forge, R. (2015). Coronary heart disease in J.S. Skinner, C.X. Bryant, S. Merrill, & D.J. Green (Eds), *American Council on Exercise medical exercise specialist manual*. San Diego, CA: American Council on Exercise.

Phelan, S., & Wing, R. R. (2005). Long-term weight loss maintenance. *The American journal of clinical nutrition, 82*(1), 222S-225S. https://doi.org/10.1093/ajcn/82.1.222S

Smith, U. (2015). Abdominal obesity: A marker of ectopic fat accumulation. *The Journal of Clinical Investigation, 125*(5), 1790-1792. https://doi.org/10.1172/JCI815

St-Onge, M. P., & Gallagher, D. (2010). Body composition changes with aging: the cause or the result of alterations in metabolic rate and macronutrient oxidation? *Nutrition, 26*(2), 152-155. https://doi.org/10.1016/j.nut.2009.07.004

Trexler, E. T., Smith-Ryan, A. E., & Norton, L. E. (2014). Metabolic adaptation to weight loss: Implications for the athlete. *Journal of the International Society of Sports Nutrition, 11*(1), 7. https://doi.org/10.1186/1550-2783-11-7

Villablanca, P. A., Alegria, J. R., Mookadam, F., Holmes, D. R., Jr., Wright, R. S., & Levine, J. A. (2015). Nonexercise activity thermogenesis in obesity management. *Mayo Clinic Proceedings, 90*(4), 509-519. https://doi.org/10.1016/j.mayocp.2015.02.001

Waters, H., & Graf, M. (2018). *The cost of chronic diseases in the U.S.: Executive summary*. Washington, DC: Milken Institute.

CHAPTER 13 METABOLIC SYNDROME

By the end of this chapter you will understand:

- Characteristics and diagnostic criteria
- Treatment strategies
  - o Pharmacological
  - o Nutrition
  - o Activity
- Comorbidities and associations
- Risks and contraindications
- FITT

Characteristics

Originally introduced in the 1920s, Metabolic Syndrome (MetS) did not gain attention until 1998 when the World Health Organization provided a first definition. A final definition was agreed upon in 2005: Metabolic syndrome is a cluster of risk factors that, in concert, increase the threat for developing cardiovascular disease and Type II diabetes (T2DM) (Kaur, 2014). The consequences of MetS is increased insulin resistance, low grade systemic inflammation, elevated HTN, and a pro-thrombotic state. Risk factors are listed below, and for a diagnosis of MetS an individual must have three risk factors or more (Kaur, 2014; Sorace, Ronai, & Churilla, 2014):

- Abdominal obesity as indicated by a waist circumference of ≥40” for men or ≥35” for women.

- Triglyceride levels of ≥150 mg/dl.
- HDL levels of <40 mg/dl for men and <50 mg/dl for women.
- Blood pressure ≥ 130/85 mm/Hg.
- Fasting glucose level of ≥100 mg/dl.

The incidence of MetS has increased in tandem with the incidences of obesity and T2DM; as of 2012, one-third of U.S. adults met the criteria for MetS (Moore, Chaudhary, & Akinyemiju, 2017; Saklayen, 2018). Consequently, an individual with MetS is twice as likely to develop cardiovascular disease (CVD) in the next 10 years, and 5-10 times as likely to develop type II diabetes (Franklin, Miller,& McCullough, 2015; Cornier et al., 2008). A client diagnosed with MetS, based on the CVD risk factors listed in Table 2.2, and the results from a physical activity risk stratification form, may meet the criteria for high risk, and should be treated accordingly.

The underlying cause of MetS is adipose tissue. Macrophages are large white blood cells in various tissues of the body. When stored in adipose tissue, the accumulation of macrophages cause, in part, metabolic dysregulation and a chronic state of low-grade inflammation (Moore, et al., 2017; Russo & Lumeng, 2018; Saklayen, 2018). Systemic inflammation can impair endothelial function, lead to blood clots, and CVD. Additionally, adipocytes, the cells that store fat and make up adipose tissue, secrete numerous hormones. The hormone leptin suppresses appetite and facilitates energy intake when energy stores are low. Conversely, the absence of leptin can result in extreme obesity. The hormone adiponectin regulates triglyceride and glucose metabolism by increasing insulin sensitivity, decreasing the size of adipocytes, and increasing mitochondrial density (Saklayen, 2018). Ghrelin, a hormone in the gut, is responsible for triggering satiety. Ghrelin increases during hunger and decreases after food intake. Weight loss also increases ghrelin that may cause individuals who are dieting trouble with continued weight loss (Franklin, et al., 2015).

Treatment Strategies

Nutrition

The most effective treatment for MetS is lifestyle change (Franklin et al., 2015; Kaur, 2014). Effective interventions are weight management via diet and exercise, and clinical intervention. Nutritional advice should be given only by a registered dietician or a physician with education and experience in nutritional counseling. However, general guidelines are:

- A daily deficit of 500-750 calories.
- Restrict certain high glycemic foods.
- Increase daily fiber consumption.
- Reduce saturated fats.
- Reduce simple sugars.
- Increase legumes and whole grains.

Pharmacology and surgery

A realistic expectation is for a reduction of 7-10% of bodyweight in 6-12-months. Any intervention needs to account for individuality and adherence (Franklin et al., 2015). Clinical interventions include weight loss drugs, bariatric surgery, and when appropriate, pharmacological treatment for individual risk factors. Pharmacological treatments will usually address one or more of the underlying diseases rather than the cluster of diseases that make up MetS. Accordingly, a CXS should be aware of any side effects of a prescribed medication.

Activity

The chances of developing MetS is almost double for individuals who perform no moderate or vigorous activity compared to individuals who meet or exceed the recommended guideline of 150 minutes per week (Cornier et al., 2008). Physical activity and obesity are generally inversely related; however, chronic inflammation often associated with chronic pain can be reduced with physical activity without weight loss (Paley & Johnson, 2016). In addition to expending calories and increasing lean body mass and RMR, resistance training can alleviate risk factors associated with the components of MetS, including lower cholesterol and triglycerides, help with glycemic control and insulin sensitivity, lower blood pressure, and reduced central and total adiposity (Sorace et al., 2014). There is also evidence that participation in resistance exercise, even in small doses and independent of aerobic exercise, is associated with a lower risk of ever developing MetS (Bakker et al., 2017). Aerobic exercise has been demonstrated to reduce adipose tissue hypoxia and increase vascularization, partially via a reduction of arterial stiffness, allowing for better blood flow and increased tissue oxygenation (Donley et al., 2014; Paley & Johnson, 2016). Aerobic exercise is associated with a reduction of pain related to chronic low-grade inflammation, a decrease in mechanical loading, better sleep, and fewer depressive symptoms. Flexibility, balance, and neuromuscular control may be negatively affected in clients with MetS (Chang et al., 2015); therefore integrating flexibility and neuromuscular training into an exercise program may be beneficial.

Unfortunately, due to the cluster of diseases associated with MetS, it is difficult to develop one exercise plan to accommodate all risk factors. Therefore, it is often advised a client diagnosed with MetS to seek a medically supervised exercise program. However, if a client with MetS has a medical release to exercise, the best results are achieved through a combination of resistance and aerobic exercise. Furthermore, recent evidence suggests an increase in physical activity with an emphasis on high intensity interval training may produce the greatest results for fat reduction and an increase in lean tissue (Paley & Johnson, 2018).

Cardiovascular exercise can be performed 5 or more days per week, with an RPE of 11-13, gradually increasing to 60 minutes per day (Franklin et al., 2015). Resistance training can be performed 2x per week, starting with a single set for each major muscle group with an intensity of 40% 1RM, with a gradual increase to multiple sets with an intensity of 80% 1RM (Sorace et al., 2014). FITT guidelines for MetS are detailed in Table 13.1.

Keep in mind contraindications for each component of MetS should be considered independently.

Table 13.1

FITT guidelines for metabolic syndrome

Mode	Frequency	Intensity	Time	Type
Aerobic	≥ 5 days/week to maximize caloric expenditure	40-60% HRR with RPE 11-13	30 min/day with a goal of reaching 60 min/day limited capacity: 3-6 10 min bouts/day to accumulate 30-60min/day	Rhythmic activities that target large muscle groups
Resistance—same as healthy adults	Each major muscle group 2-3 days/week	60%–70% of the 1RM (moderate to hard intensity) for novice to intermediate exercisers ≥80% of the 1RM (hard to very high intensity) for experienced strength trainers <50% of the 1RM for muscular endurance	8-12 exercises 8–12 reps to improve strength 15–20 reps to improve muscular endurance 2-4 sets	Resistance exercises involving each major muscle group, targeting larger groups first
Flexibility same as healthy adults	≥ 2-3 days/week	Stretch to the point of feeling tightness or slight discomfort	Static stretching hold for 10-30 sec. or up to 60 sec. for older individuals For PNF stretching, a 3- to 6-sec contraction at 20%–75% maximum voluntary contraction followed by a 10-30 sec. assisted stretch	Static flexibility, Dynamic flexibility PNF
Neuromuscular exercise training same as healthy adults	≥2-3 days/week	N/A	≥20-30 min/bout	Exercise that challenges motor skills, coordination, and proprioception such as Yoga or Tai Chi

Franklin et al., 2015; Sorace et al., 2014

Discussion and application

1. What is Metabolic Syndrome and what are it's associated conditions?
2. Why is exercise an important component of treating MetS?

References

Bakker, E. A., Lee, D. C., Sui, X., Artero, E. G., Ruiz, J. R., Eijsvogels, T. M.,...& Blair, S. N. (2017). Association of resistance exercise, independent of and combined with aerobic exercise, with the incidence of metabolic syndrome. *Mayo Clinic Proceedings, 92*(8), 1214-1222. Elsevier. https://doi.org/10.1016/j.mayocp.2017.02.018

Chang, K. V., Hung, C. Y., Li, C. M., Lin, Y. H., Wang, T. G., Tsai, K. S., & Han, D. S. (2015). Reduced flexibility associated with metabolic syndrome in community-dwelling elders. *PLoS One, 10*(1), e0117167. https://doi.org/10.1371/journal.pone.0117167

Cornier, M. A., Dabelea, D., Hernandez, T. L., Lindstrom, R. C., Steig, A. J., Stob, N. R.,...Eckel, R. H. (2008). The metabolic syndrome. *Endocrine Review, 29*(7), 777-822. https://doi.org/10.1210/er.2008-0024

Donley, D. A., Fournier, S. B., Reger, B. L., DeVallance, E., Bonner, D. E., Olfert, I. M.,...Chantler, P. D. (2014). Aerobic exercise training reduces arterial stiffness in metabolic syndrome. *Journal of Applied Physiology, 116*(11), 1396-1404. https://doi.org/10.1152/japplphysiol.00151.2014

Franklin, B. A., Miller, W. M., & McCullough, P. A. (2015). The metabolic syndrome in J.S. Skinner, C.X. Bryant, S. Merrill, & D.J. Green (Eds), *American Council on Exercise medical exercise specialist manual.* San Diego, CA: American Council on Exercise

Kaur, J. (2014). A comprehensive review on metabolic syndrome. *Cardiology Research and Practice, 2014*, 943162. https://doi.org/10.1155/2014/943162

Moore, J. X., Chaudhary, N., & Akinyemiju, T. (2017). Metabolic syndrome prevalence by race/ethnicity and sex in the United States national health and nutrition examination survey, 1988-2012. *Preventing Chronic Disease, 14*, E24. https://doi.org/10.5888/pcd14.160287

Paley, C. A., & Johnson, M. I. (2016). Physical activity to reduce systemic inflammation associated with chronic pain and obesity: A narrative review. *The Clinical Journal of Pain, 32*(4), 365-370. https://doi.org/10.1097/AJP.0000000000000258

Paley, C. A., & Johnson, M. I. (2018). Abdominal obesity and metabolic syndrome: Exercise as medicine? *BMC Sports Science, Medicine and Rehabilitation, 10*, 7. https://doi.org/10.1186/s13102-018-0097-1

Russo, L., & Lumeng, C. N. (2018). Properties and functions of adipose tissue macrophages in obesity. *Immunology, 155*(4), 407-417. https://doi.org/10.1111/imm.13002

Saklayen, M. G. (2018). The global epidemic of the metabolic syndrome. *Current Hypertension Reports, 20*(2), 12. https://doi.org/10.1007/s11906-018-0812-z

Sorace, P., Ronai, P., & Churilla, J. R. (2014). Resistance training and metabolic syndrome: Muscles do matter. *ACSM's Health & Fitness Journal, 18*(6), 24-29. https://doi.org/10.1249/FIT.0000000000000074

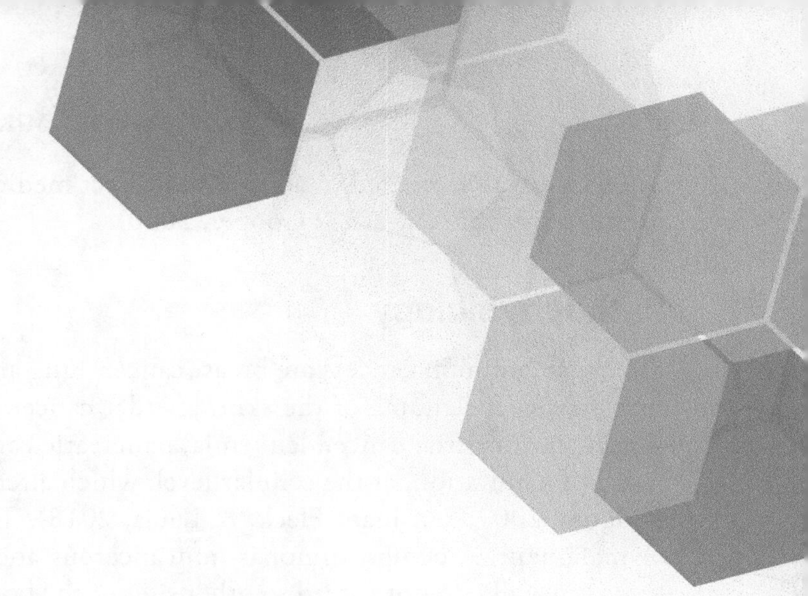

CHAPTER 14
CANCER

By the end of this chapter you will understand:

- Types and pathophysiology
- Classification
- Pharmacology
- Side effects
    - o Lymphedema
    - o Cancer-related fatigue
- Comorbidities
- Modifiable factors
    - o Nutrition
    - o Activity
    - o Exercise guidelines
    - o Considerations to exercise

Chances are you or someone you know has, or has had cancer, as it is a leading cause of death worldwide. There are almost 2 million new cases of cancer diagnosed each year in the United States and more than 600,000 people die from cancer annually (National Cancer Institute, n.d.b). In 2016, there were over 15 million cancer survivors; a number that is expected to increase to more than 20 million by 2026. Because there are more than 100 types of cancer, direct medical expenses are difficult to determine, but in 2015 it was estimated in addition to direct medical expenses, over $94 billion was lost in wages and productivity (Baxter, 2019; Cooper, 2000).

Pathophysiology

The most common cancers are breast cancer, lung and bronchus cancer, prostate cancer, colon and rectum cancer, melanoma of the skin, bladder cancer, non-Hodgkin lymphoma, kidney and renal pelvis cancer, endometrial cancer, leukemia, pancreatic cancer, thyroid cancer, and liver cancer. Cancer is the result of a mutation, at the cellular level, which alters DNA and leads to uncontrolled cell proliferation (Cooper, 2009; San Juan, Fleck, & Lucia, 2018). The mutation leads to a tumor that is either benign or malignant. A benign tumor is noncancerous and can be classified by location or cell type. Benign tumors usually do not spread to other sites of the body and do not invade surrounding tissue. Examples of benign tumors are lipomas which grow from fat cells, myomas grow from muscle or in the walls of blood vessels, fibroids grow in fibrous tissue, moles grow on the skin, and polyps grow in or on the liver. Although these are considered benign tumors, some, such as moles and polyps, can grow into cancer (Cooper, 2009).

Only malignant tumors are referred to as cancer. Malignant tumors invade surrounding tissue and spread thorough out the body via the lymphatic or circulatory system. The spreading of cancerous cells is known as metastasis. It is the spread of malignant cells in the body that makes cancer dangerous and difficult to treat (Cooper, 2009).

Classification

The classification and staging of cancer are used as a factor for diagnosis and treatment. One of the most widely used codifying systems is tumor-node-metastasis (TNM), as maintained by the American Joint Committee on Cancer and the International Union for Cancer Control (Edge & Compton, 2010). Tumor (T) describes the size and location of the main, or primary tumor, and if it has invaded surrounding tissue or organs. Node (N) indicates if cancer has infected nearby lymph nodes, and metastasis (M) indicates if cancer has spread to other parts of the body (National Cancer Institute, n.d.a). Ranking is as follows:

- T_X indicates the tumor cannot be measuredT_0 indicates no tumor; T_4 indicates invasion of a vital organ.
- N_X indicates the spread cannot be determined; N_0 indicates the tumor has not spread to any lymph nodes; N_3 indicates extensive spreading.
- M_X indicates metastasis cannot be measured; M_0 indicates no metastasis; M_1 indicates metastasis.

TNM definitions are used to stage a cancer. Stage 0 indicates abnormal cells that have not spread. Stages I-III indicate the presence of cancer; the higher the number, the larger the cancer tumor and the more it has spread into nearby tissues. Stage IV indicates a cancer has metastasized to other parts of the body (National Cancer Institute, n.d.a).

Pharmacology

Once TNM and/or stage is determined, a treatment plan is developed. Treatments usually consist of pharmacological therapy or surgery (San Juan et al., 2018). Radiation therapy attacks mutated cells by delivering high energy particles to break apart the DNA of the cell. Radiation treatments can be very precise, and target just the tumor leaving the surrounding, healthy tissue undamaged. Chemotherapy drugs involve powerful chemicals that aggressively kill cells and interfere with tumor growth by inhibiting DNA or RNA, or interfering with cell replication. Unlike other treatments, chemotherapy does not differentiate between mutated and healthy cells, and therefore often damages fast-growing healthy cells such as skin, hair, intestines, and bone marrow. Chemotherapy can be used to cure cancer, prevent recurrence of cancer, shrink tumors in preparation for other therapies, or ease symptoms. Immunotherapy and biotherapy use protein molecules to disrupt cancer cell growth while encouraging growth of healthy cells. Immuno- and biotherapies are used to fight cancer, slow the growth of mutated cells, and repair damage caused by other forms of treatment (San Juan et al., 2018). Bone marrow transplant is usually used to treat cancer of the blood. Bone marrow transplants involve destroying infected bone marrow, and replacing it with healthy marrow from a donor, or marrow taken at a time of remission. Hormone treatment is used to disrupt the growth of hormone receptor positive tumors. Hormone treatment is most thought of for breast and prostate cancers but can also be used for other cancers (San Juan et al., 2018).

Unfortunately, all of the treatments have side-effects based on the type, length, and intensity of treatment. Early side effects are nausea, vomiting, hair loss, and fatigue. More severe complications can include blood and lung embolisms, allergic reactions, and infections. Long-term side effects mostly involve toxicity that result in anemia, immunity complications, cardiovascular complications, and musculoskeletal problems that include atrophy, range of motion limitations, and osteoporosis. Neurological disorders, kidney, renal, and gastrointestinal dysfunction, and thyroid and pituitary alterations can also occur (San Juan et al., 2018).

Lymphedema

Lymphedema is a pathological dysfunction of the lymphatic system caused by damage or removal of lymph nodes allowing fluids to build and cause a harmful and painful swelling in the extremities. Some treatments, such as radiation, can cause blockage, and if cancer had spread via the lymphatic system, some nodes may need to be removed. Upper extremity lymphedema is particularly common with breast cancer, while lower extremity lymphedema is common in uterine and prostate cancers. The severity of lymphedema is dependent on how many nodes have been damaged or removed and can occur days to years after treatment or surgery.

Historically, cancer patients have been cautioned against exercise while experiencing bouts of lymphedema, however, this is not necessarily supported by research. Conversely, self-reported studies suggest resistance training may actually reduce the incidence and severity of lymphedema (San Juan, et al., 2018). It is thought physiological adaptations brought about resistance training such as increased muscle contraction and increased ventilation may be beneficial for the reduction of lymphatic fluid buildup (San Juan, et al., 2018).

Cancer Related Fatigue

Cancer-related fatigue (CRF) effects almost every cancer patient, and is defined as "a persistent, subjective sense of physical, emotional, or cognitive tiredness or exhaustion related to cancer and cancer treatment that is not proportionate to activity and interferes with normal functioning" (Blaney et al., 2010, p. 1136). CRF is the most disturbing side effect, as it can be caused by a cancer, or its treatment, or both, and can continue long term. Factors related to CRF are anxiety and depression, poor sleep and eating habits, anemia, and pain. All of these factors lead to a low level of physical activity, which leads to muscular and cardiorespiratory deconditioning, an even greater level of fatigue, and exacerbation of comorbidities.

Comorbidities

Comorbidity is the existence of a disorder or dysfunction in addition to a primary disease (Sarfati, Koczwara, & Jackson, 2016). Cancer patients with a comorbidity have higher healthcare costs, reduced survival rates, and a reduced quality of life. The most common comorbidities associated with cancer are cardiovascular disease (CVD), metabolic conditions including obesity and diabetes, and musculoskeletal dysfunction (Sarfati et al., 2016). Because of the prevalence of chronic disease associated with cancer, it is prudent a CXS understands the implications while working with a client who, in addition to cancer, has one or more chronic diseases.

There is emerging evidence suggesting cancer may be as much, if not more of a metabolic disease than a genetic disease (Coller, 2014; Seyfried, Flores, Poff, & D'Agostino, 2014). Obesity is known to increase systemic inflammation causing DNA abnormalities, as well as changes in insulin and insulin-like growth factors resulting in a favorable environment for the growth of cancer cells, particularly in adipose tissue (Doerstling, O'Flanagan, & Hursting, 2017). Obese cancer patients are also at an increased risk for CVD, secondary infection and malignancy, lymphedema, and sickness from treatments, as well as lower treatment effectiveness because of interferences with systemic delivery systems (Ligibel et al., 2014). The *Warburg effect* suggests the proliferation of some cancer cells is based on the consumption of glucose, glutamine, and glycogen that increases the circulation of insulin and promotes cellular proliferation, directly linking the biological pathway of diabetes to cancer (Coller, 2014; Sarfati et al., 2016). Combined, obesity and diabetes are linked to over a dozen types of cancer including liver, pancreas, endometrium, colorectal, breast, bladder, thyroid, and ovarian (Centers for Disease Control and Prevention, 2017; Giovannucc et al., 2010).

Modifiable Factors

Modifiable behaviors associated with cancer are weight control, diet, physical activity, exposure to tobacco products, and alcohol consumption. All except exposure to tobacco products relate directly to energy balance. Energy balance, while optimally maintained has been associated with primary prevention of cancer and increased survival rates following treatment. Obesity is second only to smoking as a modifiable risk factor for cancer (Ligibel et al., 2014). Additionally, because diabetes and obesity are two of three risk factors needed for diagnosis of metabolic syndrome (MetS) (see Chapter 13 for more information on MetS), it is important for a CXS to understand the intricacies of working with clients who have diabetes, are obese, or have the risk factors for MetS.

Similar to other chronic conditions, staying active and eating well can reduce the lifetime risk for developing cancer (Kushi et al., 2012). Due to the complexity of cancer and the intricacies of nutrition, developing healthy eating guidelines is difficult. Accordingly, the type of study, the length and scope of the study, the type of cancer, nutrient and pharmacological interaction, and dose and timing of nutrient consumption need to be considered. Individuals who want to maintain a healthy weight should consider a 50-100 calorie/day deficit, while individuals who want to lose weight should strive for a 500 calorie/day deficit (Kushi et al., 2012).

Nutrition

The American Cancer Society Guidelines for Nutrition are below (Kushi et al., 2012), and Table 14.1 lists specific nutrients that can significantly modify cancer risk and progression.

- Be as lean as possible throughout life.
- Avoid excess weight gain.
- Individuals who are currently overweight should consider losing a small amount for health benefits.
- Limit high calorie food and beverages.
- Consume a healthy diet emphasizing on plant food.
- Limit consumption of processed meat and red meat.
- Eat at least 2.5 cups of vegetables per day.
- Choose whole grains over refined grains.
- Limit alcohol consumption (1 drink/day for women, 2 drinks/day for men).

Table 14.1

Nutrients that can significantly modify cancer risk and progression

Nutrient	Effect/Benefits	Sources
Capsaicin	Helps the TRPV1 receptor, anti-inflammatory, and may induce apoptosis in non-small cell lung cancer cells, T-cell leukemia cells, esophageal carcinoma cells, astroglioma cells, and prostate, colon, and gastric cancer cells	
Ellagic Acid	May slow tumor growth	Pomegranates, grapes, walnuts, cranberries, strawberries, raspberries
Green Tea Catechins	Antioxidant capacity, anti-angiogenic, anti-mutagenic, anti-inflammatory, induction of apoptosis and cell cycle arrest that interfere with multiple signaling cascades	Green Tea
Omega 3 fatty acids	Anti-inflammatory that may slow the growth of various types of cancers including lung, colon, mammary, and prostate, and may help improve the effectiveness of various pharmacological interventions	canola oil, flaxseed, soybean, green vegetables, various fish, and fish oils
Isothiocyanates (ITCs)	Certain ITCs may help in the prevention of breast, lung, and prostate cancers. Some may also contain chemotherapeutic properties that may target cellular pathways to inhibit growth, induce apoptosis, and prevent migration	Broccoli, cauliflower, garden cress, watercress, and cabbage

Resveratrol	May inhibit the growth and development of some cancers including pancreatic, prostate, brain and esophagus	Red wine (by far the highest concentration), peanuts, blueberries
Retinoid (Vitamin A)	Inhibits cellular proliferation, induces apoptosis, cell cycle arrest, and differentiation	Cod liver oil, eggs, orange and yellow vegetables and fruits, broccoli, spinach, and most dark green, leafy vegetables

Kushi et al., 2012; Niles, & Claudio, 2012

It is beyond the scope of practice for a CXS to offer a prescriptive diet or meal plan.

Physical Activity

Physical activity is one of the modifiable risk factors in the prevention and treatment of cancer, and should be considered as part of an overall behavior modification plan, and as a cost effective means in the primary prevention of cancer (Brown, Winters-Stone, Lee, & Schmitz, 2012). The goal of exercise for cancer patients and survivors is to regain and improve physical function, aerobic capacity, strength, and flexibility. The purpose is to improve cardiorespiratory, endocrine, neurological, muscular, cognitive, and psychosocial outcomes, to reduce or delay recurrence. While it is not possible to address all of the details associated with each kind of cancer, and is well beyond the scope of this text, understanding general guidelines is essential for a CXS who works with clients who have or have had cancer. Due to the number of variables involved with a cancer diagnosis, there is no consensus for exercise recommendations. However, the American College of Sports Medicine recommends maintaining or increasing muscle mass for cancer patients; decreasing body fat and weight loss is dependent on the current status of a patient, and the type and location of cancer (Schmitz et al., 2010). The FITT guidelines for cancer (Table 14.2) are compiled from the most current data available. Each client needs to be independently evaluated and an exercise program should be based on current ability, the type and location of cancer, and the type of treatment. Furthermore, a CXS who works with cancer patients is strongly encouraged to research the specifics of the type of cancer, as well as the diagnosis and treatment plan of a client.

Table 14.2

FITT guidelines for cancer prevention, treatment, and recovery

	Frequency	Intensity	Type	Time
Aerobic exercise	Starting at 3 days/week Progressing to 5-4 days/week	40% HRR progressing to 70-85% HRR	Start with walking and add in different modalities as tolerated	10-15 min progressing to 30-45 min, or 150 min/week
Resistance training	Start at 2x/week and progress to 3x/week	30%1RM progressing to 70-80% 1RM	Start with bands, progress to machines, dumbbells, and free weights	Begin with one set and one exercise for each major muscle groups and progress to 8-10 exercises and 2-3 sets
Flexibility	Stop before discomfort or pain	As many days as possible	2-4 sets/muscle group	10-30 second static stretch

Brown et al., 2012; San Juan et al., 2018; Schmitz et al., 2010

Considerations

The following are precautions and considerations to exercise for cancer patients (San Juan et al., 2018):

- For each of the following conditions avoid or postpone exercise, but encourage performing ADLs:
    - o Temperature of > 104
    - o Anemia
    - o Low white blood cell count (neutropenia)
    - o Low platelet count (thrombocytopenia)
    - o Extreme weight loss or atrophy (cachexia)
    - o Cardiotoxicity
- Avoid high impact or contact exercise for a client who has bone cancer or is at risk for hemorrhaging (thrombocytopenia).
- Be aware of clients who experience ataxia, dizziness, or neuropathy who may be at an increased risk for falls and fractures.
- Breast cancer patients should be cautious of lymphedema in the arm or shoulder.
- Prostate cancer survivors should be perform pelvic floor exercises.

Discussion and application

1. What are the side effects of cancer treatments and how does exercise minimize side effects?
2. What are precautions to keep in mind when working with a client who has cancer?

References

Baxter, A. (2019, July 8). Cost of cancer deaths tops $94B annually. *HealthExec*. Retrieved from https://www.healthexec.com/topics/healthcare-economics/cost-cancer-deaths-tops-94b-annually

Blaney, J., Lowe-Strong, A., Rankin, J., Campbell, A., Allen, J., & Gracey, J. (2010). The Cancer Rehabilitation Journey: Barriers to and facilitators of exercise among patients with cancer-related fatigue. *Physical Therapy, 90*(8), 1135-1147. https://doi.org/10.2522/ptj.20090278

Brown, J. C., Winters-Stone, K., Lee, A., & Schmitz, K. H. (2012). Cancer, physical activity, and exercise. *Comprehensive Physiology, 2*(4), 2775-2809. https://doi.org/10.1002/cphy.c120005

Centers for Disease Control and Prevention. (2017). About cancer: Obesity and cancer. Retrieved from https://www.cancer.gov/about-cancer/causes-prevention/risk/obesity/obesity-fact-sheet

Coller, H. A. (2014). Is cancer a metabolic disease? *The American Journal of Pathology, 184*(1), 4-17. https://doi.org/10.1016/j.ajpath.2013.07.035

Cooper, G. M. (2000). *The cell: A molecular approach* (2 ed.). Sunderland, MA: Sinauer Associates. Retrieved from https://www.ncbi.nlm.nih.gov/books/NBK9963/

Doerstling, S. S., O'Flanagan, C. H., & Hursting, S. D. (2017). Obesity and cancer metabolism: A perspective on interacting tumor-intrinsic and extrinsic factors. *Frontiers in Oncology, 7*, 216. https://doi.org/10.3389/fonc.2017.00216

Edge, S. B., & Compton, C. C. (2010). The American Joint Committee on Cancer: the 7th edition of the AJCC cancer staging manual and the future of TNM. *Annals of Surgical Oncology, 17*(6), 1471-1474. https://doi.org/10.1245/s10434-010-0985-4

Kushi, L. H., Doyle, C., McCullough, M., Rock, C. L., Demark-Wahnefried, W., Bandera, E. V.,... Physical Activity Guidelines Advisory, C. (2012). American Cancer Society guidelines on nutrition and physical activity for cancer prevention: Reducing the risk of cancer with healthy food choices and physical activity. *CA: A Cancer Journal for Clinicians, 62*(1), 30-67. https://doi.org/10.3322/caac.20140

Ligibel, J. A., Alfano, C. M., Courneya, K. S., Demark-Wahnefried, W., Burger, R. A., Chlebowski, R. T.,...Hudis, C. A. (2014). American Society of Clinical Oncology position statement on obesity and cancer. *The Journal of Clinical Oncology, 32*(31), 3568-3574. https://doi.org/1010.1200/JCO.2014.58.4680

National Cancer Institute. (n.d.a). NCI dictionary of cancer terms. Retrieved from https://www.cancer.gov/publications/dictionaries/cancer-terms/def/tnm-staging-system

National Cancer Institute. (n.d.b). Understanding cancer: Cancer statistics. Retrieved from https://www.cancer.gov/about-cancer/understanding/statistics

Niles, R. M., & Claudio, P. P. (2012). *Nutrition and cancer from epidemiology to biology*. Oak Park, Ill: Bentham Science Publishers.

San Juan, A. F., Fleck, S. J., & Lucia, A. (2018). Cancer in P.L. Jacobs (Ed) *NSCA's essentials of training special populations*. Champaign, IL: Human Kinetics.

Sarfati, D., Koczwara, B., & Jackson, C. (2016). The impact of comorbidity on cancer and its treatment. *CA: A Cancer Journals for Clinicians, 66*(4), 337-350. https://doi.org/10.3322/caac.21342

Schmitz, K. H., Courneya, K. S., Matthews, C., Demark-Wahnefried, W., Galvao, D. A., Pinto, B. M., Schwartz, A. L. (2010). American College of Sports Medicine roundtable on exercise guidelines for cancer survivors. *Medicine and Science in Sports and Exercise, 42*(7), 1409-1426. https://doi.org/10.1249/MSS.0b013e3181e0c112

Seyfried, T. N., Flores, R. E., Poff, A. M., & D'Agostino, D. P. (2014). Cancer as a metabolic disease: Implications for novel therapeutics. *Carcinogenesis, 35*(3), 515-527. https://doi.org/ 10.1093/ carcin/bgt480

CHAPTER 15
PREGNANCY

By the end of this chapter you will understand:

- Benefits of exercise before, during, and after pregnancy
- Weight gain recommendations
- Response to exercise
    - o Musculoskeletal
    - o Physiological
- Preeclampsia
- Gestational diabetes
- Diastasis recti
- Precautions and considerations for exercise
- Activity recommendations
    - o While pregnant
    - o Postpartum

Benefits of Exercise

Over the past decade, there has been mounting evidence supporting the benefits of exercise during and after pregnancy. Healthy pregnant women are encouraged to exercise to maintain a healthy weight, reduce the chance for gestational diabetes, and improve psychological well-being. Pregnant women who exercise, regardless if they exercised prior to becoming pregnant or started after, experience fewer delivery and postpartum complications, have a lower incidence of edema, and are more likely to deliver a normal size baby (American College of Sports Medicine [ACSM], 2018). To encourage prescriptive exercise during pregnancy, The American College of Obstetricians and Gynecologists (ACOG), as well as a joint Canadian task force, comprised of the Society of Obstetricians and Gynaecologists of Canada and the Canadian Society for Exercise Physiology, developed guidelines for exercise during pregnancy (ACOG, 2015; Davies, Wolfe, Mottola, & MacKinnon, 2003). They are summarized below:

- Exercise during pregnancy has minimal risks and multiple benefits.
- Exercise may need to be modified.
- A clinical evaluation should be performed prior to beginning an exercise program.
- All women without contraindications should be encouraged to participate in aerobic and strength-conditioning exercises as part of a healthy lifestyle during pregnancy.
- Reasonable goals of aerobic conditioning in pregnancy should be to maintain a good fitness level throughout pregnancy without trying to reach peak fitness or train for an athletic competition.
- Women should choose activities that minimize the risk of loss of balance and fetal trauma.
- Women should be advised that adverse pregnancy or neonatal outcomes are not higher for women who exercise.
- Initiation of pelvic floor exercises in the immediate postpartum period may reduce the risk of future urinary incontinence.
- Women should be advised that moderate exercise during lactation does not affect the quantity or composition of breast milk or effect infant growth.

Weight Gain Recommendations

The most apparent physiological change during pregnancy is weight gain, averaging 25-40 pounds, or 15-25% of pre-pregnancy weight (ACSM, 2018; Bush, 2018; Merrill, 2015). The Institute of Medicine recommends underweight women (<18 BMI) gain 28-40 pounds, normal weight women (18.8-24.9 BMI) should gain 25-35 pounds, overweight women (25-29.9BMI) should gain 15-25 pounds, and obese women (>30 BMI) should gain 11-20 pounds. Weight gains below these recommendations can result in low infant birth weight, and above these recommendations can result in fetal macrosomia (birth weight above 8lbs,13oz.), difficulty with natural birth, and trauma to the mother and baby (ACSM, 2018; Bush, 2018; Merrill, 2015). Additional weight gain can also lead to musculoskeletal problems, hypertension or preeclampsia, and gestational diabetes.

Musculoskeletal Response

During pregnancy, the musculoskeletal response includes a shifting center of gravity, increased joint forces, and pelvic girdle pain. Over 60% of pregnant women will suffer low back pain during and following pregnancy due to lordosis from weight gain, and a change in the center of gravity (COG) (ACOG, 2015). Additionally, pelvic girdle pain is experienced by 25% of pregnant women (Sarıkaya, Yılmaz,

& Okumuş, 2016). The pain often radiates from the tailbone or sacroiliac to the posterior thigh. The combination of weight gain, the COG moving forward, and excessive joint mobility caused by the release of the hormones relaxin and progesterone, often leads to joint pain and altered gait mechanics that need to be considered during activity, and for program design. Accordingly, heavy weights and activities that increase the risk of falling should be avoided (ACOG, 2015; Davies et al., 2003).

Physiological Response

In addition to changes in the musculoskeletal system, there are also changes to a woman's cardiovascular, respiratory, and thermoregulatory systems. While blood volume, heart rate, and stroke volume increase, vascular resistance decreases, resulting in lightheadedness, dizziness, and fatigue. Additionally, the change in hemodynamics can cause hypotension while in static positions such as those found in yoga, or supine positions (ACOG, 2015; ACSM, 2018). Changes in tidal volume in pressure gradients designed to increase oxygen uptake and carbon dioxide emission can cause a sense of breathlessness. Also, a decrease in pulmonary reserve may hinder anaerobic and aerobic exercise and limit the overall workload. Interestingly, women who perform aerobic exercise regularly during pregnancy often experience a training effect that increases aerobic capacity after birth (ACOG, 2015; Merrill, 2015). The increase in tidal volume and decrease in vascular resistance also permits greater blood flow to the skin and lungs, allowing better heat dissipation. To maintain positive heat balance, blood volume needs to remain high, suggesting proper hydration is critical. Furthermore, it is recommended pregnant women avoid exercising in high heat or humid conditions and wear loose fitting clothing for better air circulation (ACOG, 2015; Merrill, 2015).

Preeclampsia

Preeclampsia is persistent hypertension, and effects up to 4% of pregnant women (Merrill, 2015). Although preeclampsia can present at any time during pregnancy, it usually occurs later and sometimes even up to 6 weeks after pregnancy. Women who suffer from preeclampsia have high levels of protein in their urine and may experience edema in the extremities. Although the cause is unknown, it is thought to effect women who are overweight and have poor nutritional habits. The only cure for preeclampsia is birth. Preeclampsia risk factors, signs, and complications can be found in Table 15.1.

It is beyond the scope of a CXS to work with a client who suffers from preeclampsia.

Table 15.1

Preeclampsia risk factors, signs, and complications

Risk factors	Signs	Complications
First pregnancy	Rapid weight gain	Stroke
History of preeclampsia	Edema	Seizures
An immediate relative who suffered from preeclampsia,	Headache	Heart failure in the mother
Multiple gestations	Nausea	Impaired mental abilities in the baby
A history of diabetes, kidney disease, or some autoimmune diseases	Abdominal pain	Stunted growth for a baby
	High blood pressure	Fetal death

Merrill, 2015

Gestational Diabetes

Gestational diabetes mellitus (GDM) can affect 1 in 7 births and is characterized by exacerbated insulin resistance in pregnant women (International Diabetes Federation, 2019; Merrill, 2015). This period of hyperglycemia, or carbohydrate intolerance, usually resolves following birth (Padayachee & Coombes, 2015). Non-modifiable risk factors include ethnic minority (African American, Native American, Hispanic, and some Asians cultures), maternal age (>35), polycystic ovarian syndrome, family history of diabetes, and preeclampsia. Modifiable risk factors include obesity and poor nutrition (Padayachee & Coombes, 2015). The effects of GDM can be larger than normal birthweight, jaundice, nervous system disorders, and pulmonary distress. Babies may also suffer from hypoglycemia immediately following birth and have a greater chance for obesity or metabolic disorders. Exercise and proper nutrition prior to pregnancy can reduce the likelihood of GDM by almost 25%. Additionally, although there is no cure for GDM, the primary mode of treatment is activity and nutrition counselling. A CXS can only work with a client with GDM after a woman has received medical clearance to exercise, and often requires little to no exercise modifications as compared to healthy pregnant women.

Diastasis Recti

Another topic of concern for pregnant women is abdominal diastasis recti (ADR) (ACOG, 2015; Merrill, 2015). ADR is characterized by a separation of the right and left sides of the rectus abdominals, and is caused by mechanical stress, weak abdominal muscles, and an increase of hormones. Women with multiple gestation, who are petite, have had multiple pregnancies, or who have poor muscle tone are at risk. Symptoms include a protruding stomach, low back pain, poor posture, and constipation. There are no readily available statistics on diastasis recti, but it is thought it may affect 60-100% of pregnant women at some point during or after pregnancy. To avoid exacerbating ADR, caution should be used when performing core, abdominal, and trunk movements such as flexion, extension, or rotation. Accordingly, static abdominal exercises should be considered.

Precautions and Considerations for Exercise

Each condition, including a healthy pregnancy, should be considered when designing an exercise program for pregnant women, women who are trying to get pregnant, or women who have already given birth. The PARmed-X (physical activity readiness questionnaire for pregnant women developed by the Canadian Society for Exercise Physiologists), or a similar tool should be filled out by potentially pregnant clients. The following are precautions and recommendations for exercise during pregnancy (ACSM, 2018; Merrill, 2015):

- Women not previously active should begin slowly and progress.
- Pregnancy alters the heart rate response, so the RPE scale or talk test should be used to gauge intensity.
- Exercise programs should include aerobic and resistance training, stretching, and a 15-minute warm up and cool down period.
- An additional 300 calories/day may be needed to account for the caloric needs of the baby.
- Exercise should be performed in a cool, dry environment.

- Maintain hydration by consuming a pint of water prior to exercise, and a cup of water every 20 minutes during exercise.
- Avoid static positions and exercises performed in a supine position.
- Due to joint laxity, joints may be prone to injury.
- Avoid the Valsalva maneuver.
- Avoid high risk activities that may result in fetal damage due to contact, falling, or oxygen deprivation:
    - o Snow and water skiing
    - o Rock climbing
    - o Scuba diving
    - o High altitude adventures
    - o Horseback riding
    - o Contact sports

Table 15.2 lists contraindications to exercise while pregnant, and warning signs when to immediately stop exercise and seek medical attention. A relative contraindication suggests the benefits of exercise may not outweigh the risks of exercise and each risk needs to be individually considered, while an absolute contraindication could cause injury, harm, or death (Davies, et al., 2003). Women who were active prior to pregnancy, and have no complications, should follow the exercise guidelines for apparently healthy adults during pregnancy, and postpartum. Women who were not active prior to pregnancy should avoid high intensity exercise. Regardless, pregnant women should engage in at least 30 minutes of light to moderate intensity exercise most days of the week for a total of 150 minutes per week. Guidelines for intensity have been developed based on BMI and age; moderate intensity is recommended for women with a BMI of <25, and light intensity for women with a BMI of >25 (Merrill, 2015). Table 15.3 provides exercise guidelines for pregnant women.

Table 15.2

Contraindications and warning signs for exercise during pregnancy

Relative contraindications	Absolute contraindications	Warning sings to stop exercise
Anemia	Hemodynamically significant heart disease	Vaginal bleeding
Maternal cardiac arrhythmia	Restrictive lung disease	Painful contractions
Chronic bronchitis	Incompetent cervix	Amniotic fluid leakage
Morbid obesity or extreme underweight	Multiple gestations	Dyspnea before exertion
Eating disorder	Persistent bleeding	Dizziness
Orthopedic limitations	Placenta previa after week 26	Headache
Heavy smoker	Premature labor	Angina
Previous spontaneous abortion	Ruptured membranes	Poor balance
Previous preterm birth	Uncontrolled type I diabetes	Calf pain or swelling

Poorly controlled type 1 diabetes	Uncontrolled thyroid disease	Decreased fetal movement
Poorly controlled hypertension	Uncontrolled CVD	
Comorbidities	Preeclampsia	
	Severe anemia	

ACOG, 2015; Bush, 2018; Davies et al., 2003

Table 15.3

Exercise recommendations for pregnant women

	Frequency	Intensity	Time	Type
Aerobic	3-5days/week	RPE 12-14, or somewhat difficult BMI <25: 40-60% HRR BMI>25: <40%HRR	At least 150 min/ week 120 min. Active 15 min. warm up 15 min. cool down	Lower skill level balance activities: • Walking • Swimming • Stationary cycle • Low impact aerobics
Resistance	2-3 days/week	Relatively low weights: 40-60% 1RM or 60-80% of 10 rep max	12 reps/set 12-15 reps/set after week 28	All modalities • Controlled ROM • Focus on postural muscles, particularly in the later stages of pregnancy • Nothing supine (after 1st trimester) • No isometrics • Avoid Valsalva maneuver
Flexibility	Daily	Below discomfort level	Static stretch hold for 10-30 sec.	Be aware of joint and ligament laxity Avoid ballistic stretching
Kegels-prenatal	Daily		10 reps Hold for 3 seconds	
Kegels-postpartum	3x/day		10 reps Contract for 10 sec Relax for 10 sec	

ACOG, 2015; ACSM, 2018, Bush, 2018; Davies et al., 2018

Postpartum Exercise Recommendations

There is no timeline defining the postpartum period; however, most physiological and morphological changes continue for 4-6 weeks after birth (Evenson, Mottola, Owe, Rousham, & Brown, 2014). The ACOG suggests pre-pregnancy levels of activity can resume as soon as it is medically safe, based on physician approval. The benefits of postpartum activity are similar to benefits from prenatal activity; improved cardiorespiratory and muscular fitness, improved mood, and weight management. The goal of exercise following birth is to have some personal time and regain a sense of control. Unfortunately, women who do not resume activity postpartum often stay inactive for years (Evenson et al., 2014). Assuming no complications immediately following birth, mild exercise to include walking, pelvic floor exercises, and light stretching can be performed. Kegels can help with postpartum recovery, decrease urinary incontinence, and pelvic floor muscle function. Postpartum posture also needs to be considered. Added body weight, carrying a newborn, and carrying and moving equipment designed for an infant, can lead to an anterior posture indicated by rounded shoulders, upper cross syndrome, and kyphosis. Stretching the pectorals and the shoulder girdle, and strengthening the scapula and neck may be appropriate to improve posture and relive low back pain. The following suggestions can reacclimate a client to activity (Merrill, 2015):

- Begin slowly.
- Avoid excessive fatigue.
- Support and compress the abdomen and breasts.
- Stop activity when it hurts.

Discussion and application

1. Describe the physiological changes that takes place in females during pregnancy and how those changes will effect exercise program design.
2. What elements should be considered in an exercise program for post-partum women and why?

References

American College of Obstetricians and Gynecologists. (2015). Physical activity and exercise during pregnancy and the postpartum period. Committee Opinion No. 650. *Obstetrics and Gynecology, 126*(6), e135-142. Retrieved from https://www.acog.org/Resources-And-Publications/Committee-Opinions/Committee-on-Obstetric-Practice/Physical-Activity-and-Exercise-During-Pregnancy-and-the-Postpartum-Period

American College of Sports Medicine. (2018). *ACSM's resources for the exercise physiologist: A practical guide for the health fitness professional* (P. Magyari, R. Lite, M. W. Kilpatrick, & J. E. Schoffstall Eds. 2 ed.). Philadelphia, PA: Wolters Kluwer.

Bush, J. A. (2018). Female specific conditions in P.L. Jacobs (Ed) *NSCA's essentials of training special populations.* Champaign, IL: Human Kinetics.

Davies, G. A. L., Wolfe, L. A., Mottola, M. F., & MacKinnon, C. (2003). Joint SOGC/CSEP clinical practice guideline: Exercise in pregnancy and the postpartum period. *Canadian Journal of Applied Physiology, 28*(3), 329-341. https://doi.org/10.1139/h03-024

Evenson, K. R., Mottola, M. F., Owe, K. M., Rousham, E. K., & Brown, W. J. (2014). Summary of international guidelines for physical activity after pregnancy. *Obstetrical & Gynecological Survey, 69*(7), 407-414. https://doi.org/10.1097/OGX.0000000000000077

International Diabetes Federation. (2019). Care and prevention: Gestational diabetes. Retrieved from https://www.idf.org/our-activities/care-prevention/gdm

Merrill, S. (2015). Prenatal and postpartum exercise in J.S. Skinner, C.X. Bryant, S. Merrill, & D.J. Green (Eds), *American Council on Exercise medical exercise specialist manual.* San Diego, CA: American Council on Exercise.

Padayachee, C., & Coombes, J. S. (2015). Exercise guidelines for gestational diabetes mellitus. *World Journal of Diabetes, 6(*8), 1033-1044. https://doi.org/10.4239/wjd.v6.i8.1033

Sarikaya, E., Yılmaz, S., & Okumuş, M. (2016). Pregnancy-related pelvic girdle pain. *Gynecology Obstetrics & Reproductive Medicine, 20*(2), 122-125. Retrieved from http://gorm.com.tr/index.php/GORM

CHAPTER 16
CORE, BALANCE, AND GAIT

By the end of this chapter you will understand:

- Movement and stability
- Postural control
  - Static balance
  - Dynamic balance
- The importance of core strength for balance and movement
- Core anatomy
  - Musculature
  - Fascial subsystems
- Gait mechanics
- Exercise strategies

Movement and Stability

As mentioned in Chapter 4, the first goal of any training program is to ensure activities of daily living (ADLs) can be performed. Each foundational functional movement (squatting, single leg movements such as lunges or walking, pushing, pulling, and rotating [Cook, Burton, & Hoogenboom, 2006; Galati, 2015]) requires a certain level of stability and mobility through the kinetic chain. Stability is the body's ability to resist a change of direction and is achieved via muscle activation that creates stiffness around a joint; mobility indicates the extent of articulation around a joint (Comana & McGrath, 2015; Galati,

2015). For static and dynamic balance to be achieved, and proprioception to be effective, each joint or segment needs to be able to perform its primary function as listed below and detailed in Figure 4.2.

- Feet—stability
- Ankles—mobility
- Knees—stability
- Hips—mobility
- Lumbar spine—stability
- Thoracic spine—mobility
- Scapula—stability
- Glenohumeral—mobility

Postural Control

For ADLs to be performed, proper movement and postural control are required; however, in addition to joint mobility and stability, proper movement and postural control also require static and dynamic balance. Balance involves the integration of nervous signals from the proprioceptive, vestibular, and visual systems. Static balance is characterized by an ability to maintain the body's center of gravity (COG) over its base of support (BOS) (Dalcourt & Comana, 2015; Wang, Ji, Jiang, Liu, & Jiao, 2016). The COG is the point at which all weight is evenly distributed around and may change as the body is repositioned. The base of support is the area around and between the points of a body in contact with a surface. The proprioceptive system provides information regarding spatial relationships and movement, the vestibular system (inner ear balance mechanism) provides information regarding inertia and acceleration, and the visual system provides information regarding layout and location, and accounts for up to 75% of human sensory input (Dalcourt & Comana, 2015).

Dynamic balance is the ability to maintain postural control while moving and involves internal and external input to maintain postural control when stability is disrupted. Based on neuromuscular control, the body-brain connection uses three movement strategies to maintain postural control and stabilize the COG during deliberate and unplanned disturbances to stability (Dalcourt & Comana, 2015; Horak, 2006). When there is a small disturbance, postural sway will occur primarily at the ankle, allowing the COG to remain over the BOS. For disturbances of a larger or faster magnitude, the postural sway initiates at the hips allowing the upper and lower body to move in opposite directions. The third strategy involves the knee or taking a step. This is usually initiated when ankle and hip strategies are insufficient to retain the COG over the BOS, or when purposeful dynamic balance occurs such as walking (Horak, 2006). Each strategy exemplifies Newton's third law of motion; for every action there is an equal and opposite reaction. When balance is disturbed, an equal reaction takes place in the form of postural sway or stepping.

The Core

The purpose of the core in the kinetic chain is to provide stability for efficient movement. Based on the three movement strategies for balance, and because all movement passes through the core to the extremities, it is easy to see how important the core and its subsystems are for balance. The core, also known as the lumbo-pelvic-hip complex, has 29 pairs of muscles to stabilize the spine and pelvis for static balance, and stabilize the kinetic chain for dynamic balance and efficient movement (Faries & Greenwood, 2007). The core is a box with the diaphragm at the top and the pelvic floor at the bottom. Abdominal, paraspinal, and gluteal muscles are in the front and back, and oblique muscles make up the sides (Huxel-Bliven & Anderson, 2013). The synergistic relationship between the mobilizers and stabilizers of the core allows movement to be transferred from one extremity to another.

In addition to the core, there are four fascial subsystems, or slings, that transfer kinetic energy from one part of the body to another and assist in load transfer between the upper and lower body (Dalcourt & Comana, 2015; Donatelli, 2007). A fifth sub-system, known as the serape effect, provides stability and torque production during rotational movements by crisscrossing certain segments of the body (Santana, McGill, & Brown, 2015). Table 16.1 details the muscles and fascia associated with each sling.

Table 16.1

Muscles and fascia associated with myofascial slings

Myofascial Slings	Muscles and Fascia
Posterior oblique sling	Latissimus dorsi Gluteus maximus Thoracodorsal fascia
Anterior oblique sling	External oblique Anterior abdominal fascia Contralateral internal oblique Hip adductors
Deep longitudinal sling	Peroneals Biceps femoris Sacrotuberous ligament Deep lamina of thoracodorsal fascia Erector spinae
Lateral sling	Gluteus med/min Tensor fascia latea Lateral stabilizers of thoracopelvis region
Anterior Serape	Hip flexors Adductors Internal and external obliques Right and left serratus anterior Rhomboids
Posterior Serape	Gastrocnemius and soleus Hamstrings Glutes Latissimus dorsi Pectoralis

Donatelli, 2007; Santana, McGill, & Brown, 2015

The Gait Cycle

Walking is a single-leg movement and functional ADL, and is considered a series of controlled falls and regaining balance (Dalcourt & Comana, 2015); as such, walking requires, stability, mobility, and dynamic balance. The gait cycle consists of two steps, or one stride, and starts when the heel of one foot contacts the ground and finishes on the next ground strike with the same heel. During that time, one foot is in the stance phase and stabilizing, while the other is in the swing phase and mobilizing (Kharb,

Saini, Jain, & Dhiman, 2011). Phases of the gait cycle are in Table 16.2. For proper locomotion, mobility is required in the feet and ankles, hips, pelvis, and thoracic spine, while stability is required in the feet and hips. The stability and mobility phases of the gait cycle are listed in Table 16.3.

Table 16.2

Phases of the gait cycle

Initial contact:	
Heel strike	Floor contact is made with the heel of one foot while the other foot is in terminal stance.
Loading response	Weight is transferred to forward limb. Opposite limb begins pre-swing.
Mid-stance	One limb advances while the other limb supports the body weight.
Terminal Stance	The body is still in single-limb support. It begins with heel rise and continues until the other foot strikes the ground.
Heel-off & Pre-swing	The body moves forward as the weight is transitioned from the stance leg to the opposite leg as it prepares for the heel-off.
Swing phase:	
Initial & mid	The leg transitions from heel-off and prepares for the next heel strike.
Terminal Swing phase	One leg is in terminal stance while the other is in heel strike.

Dalcourt & Comana, 2015; Kharb et al., 2011

Table 16.3

Mobility and stability phases of the gait cycle

Body part	Stabilization	Mobility
Hips	Mid-stance, swing phase of opposite leg	Swing phase
Feet/ankles	Heel strike	Heel off
Thoracic spine		Opposite shoulder extends during swing phase
Pelvis		Counter-rotates with thoracic spine

Dalcourt & Comana, 2015; Kharb et al., 2011

Exercise Strategies

It is important to understand the relationship between stability, mobility, balance, core, myofascial slings, and gait. Without the efficient transfer of loads from one body segment to another, movement and locomotion would not be possible. Therefore, to develop an exercise program a fundamental understanding of efficient core movement and dynamic balance strategies is essential. Further, any program designed to prevent an injury or correct movement dysfunction needs to incorporate neuromuscular, endurance, and strength components to challenge balance, posture, and the core (Huxel-Bliven & Anderson, 2013).

Because spinal stability and a lower risk for injury are associated with endurance, exercise strategies for the core should focus on muscular endurance and the reeducation of faulty motor patterns prior to building strength (Faries & Greenwood, 2007). To stiffen the torso, the core relies mostly on co-contraction; therefore, any training program should encourage exercises that use all of the musculature of the core, such as abdominal bracing instead of drawing in, crunches, or torso twists (Maeo, Takahashi, Takai, & Kanehisa, 2013: McGill, 2010). Additionally, because contracting the rectus abdominis brings the rib cage and the pelvis together, a movement not generally used for dynamic function, sit-ups are discouraged. McGill (2010) suggests the following training progression below (see Chapter 22 for more details on training of the core and low back). This progression can be incorporated with the core and myofascial sling exercises listed in Table 16.4.

1. Corrective and therapeutic exercise.
2. Groove appropriate and perfect motion and motor patterns.
3. Build whole-body and joint stability (mobility at some joints such as the hips and stability through the lumbar/core region).
4. Increase endurance.
5. Build strength—for occupational/athletic clients.
6. Develop speed, power, and agility—for occupational/athletic clients.

Table 16.4

Core and myofascial sling exercises

Core stabilization and motor pattern recruitment	Diaphragmic breathing
	Abdominal Bracing
	Hollowing
	Modified curl-up—one leg straight, one leg bent
	Side bridge
	Quadruped birddog
Anterior oblique sling	Plank
	Standing cable press
	High to low cable chop
Posterior oblique sling	Quadruped birddog
	Single arm cable pull
	Single-leg Romanian deadlift
Lateral sling	Side plank
	Lateral step-up
	Lateral lunge
Deep longitudinal sling	Bridging
	Step-up
	Romanian deadlift
	Windmill
	Turkish get-up

Dalcourt & Comana, 2015; Faries & Davies, 2007, Huxel Bliven & Anderson, 2013; McGill, 2010

Static balance can be progressed by increasing the need for postural sway via manipulation of a stance used for any given exercise (Muehlbauer, Roth, Bopp, & Granacher, 2012). To further challenge balance, sensory perception can be manipulated by having a client stand on a foam pad and/or block a client's vision. The stance progression should be:

- Bi-pedal—feet next to each.
- Semi-tandem—one foot slightly in front and offline of the other.
- Tandem—one foot directly in front and inline of the other.
- Mono-pedal—single leg.
- Repeat standing on a foam pad.
- Repeat with hindered vision.

To reduce the likelihood of falling, a client should start with static balance and progress to dynamic (Dalcourt & Comana, 2015; Donath, van Dieen, & Faude, 2016). After moving through the progression suggested for static balance, a directional agility program using the movement patterns below can be implemented to improve dynamic balance.

- Forward movement
- Lateral movement
- Backwards movement
- Rotational and cross-over movements
- Curving and cutting movements

To progress, these movement patterns can be manipulated by changing direction, changing acceleration and deceleration, performing them as reactive or explosive movements, or combining the movement patterns.

Discussion and application

1. What is the role of the core in balance and gait?
    a. Discuss the ankle, hip, and step strategies for recovery of balance and gait.
    b. How would you explain this to a client who displays poor balance?
2. Design balance progression for a client and explain your exercise selection.

References

Comana, F. & McGrath, C. (2015). Posture and movement in J.S. Skinner, C.X. Bryant, S. Merrill, & D.J. Green (Eds), *American Council on Exercise medical exercise specialist manual.* San Diego, CA: American Council on Exercise.

Cook, G., Burton, L., & Hoogenboom, B. (2006). Pre-participation screening: The use of fundamental movements as an assessment of function—part 1. *North American Journal of Sports Physical Therapy, 1*(2), 62-72. Retrieved from http://www.ncbi.nlm.nih.gov/pmc/articles/PMC2953313/

Dalcourt, M., & Comana, F. (2015). Balance and gait in J.S. Skinner, C.X. Bryant, S. Merrill, & D.J. Green (Eds), *American Council on Exercise medical exercise specialist manual.* San Diego, CA: American Council on Exercise.

Donatelli, R. A. (2007). *The Anatomy and Pathophysiology of the CORE.* Sports-specific Rehabilitation, 135. St. Louis, MO: Churchill Livingstone Elsevier.

Donath, L., van Dieen, J., & Faude, O. (2016). Exercise-based fall prevention in the elderly: What about agility? *Sports Medicine, 46*(2), 143-149. https://doi.org/10.1007/s40279-015-0389-5

Faries, M. D., & Greenwood, M. (2007). Core training: Stabilizing the confusion. *Strength and Conditioning Journal, 29*(2), 10. https://doi.org/10.1519/00126548-200704000-00001

Galati, T. (2015). Applying the ACE Integrated Fitness Training model in the medical exercise setting in J.S. Skinner, C.X. Bryant, S. Merrill, & D.J. Green (Eds), *American Council on Exercise medical exercise specialist manual.* San Diego, CA: American Council on Exercise.

Horak, F. B. (2006). Postural orientation and equilibrium: what do we need to know about neural control of balance to prevent falls? *Age and Ageing, 35* Suppl 2, ii7-ii11. https://doi.org/10.1093/ageing/afl077

Huxel Bliven, K. C., & Anderson, B. E. (2013). Core stability training for injury prevention. *Sports Health, 5*(6), 514-522. https://doi.org/10.1177/1941738113481200

Kharb, A., Saini, V., Jain, Y., & Dhiman, S. (2011). A review of gait cycle and its parameters. *IJCEM International Journal of Computational Engineering & Management, 13,* 78-83. Retrieved from https://www.ijcem.org/papers72011/72011_14.pdf

Muehlbauer, T., Roth, R., Bopp, M., & Granacher, U. (2012). An exercise sequence for progression in balance training. *Journal of Strength and Conditioning Research, 26*(2), 568-574. https://doi.org/10.1519/JSC.0b013e318225f3c4

Maeo, S., Takahashi, T., Takai, Y., & Kanehisa, H. (2013). Trunk muscle activities during abdominal bracing: Comparison among muscles and exercises. *Journal of Sports Science and Medicine, 12*(3), 467-474. Retrieved from http://www.jssm.org

McGill, S. M. (2010). Core training: Evidence translating to better performance and injury prevention. *Strength & Conditioning Journal, 32*(3), 33-46. https://doi.org/10.1519/SSC.0b013e3181df4521

Santana, J. C., McGill, S. M., & Brown, L. E. (2015). Anterior and posterior serape: The rotational core. *Strength & Conditioning Journal, 37*(5), 8-13. https://doi.org/10.1519/SSC.0000000000000162

Wang, H., Ji, Z., Jiang, G., Liu, W., & Jiao, X. (2016). Correlation among proprioception, muscle strength, and balance. *The Journal of Physical Therapy Science, 28,* 3468–3472. https://doi.org/10.1589/jpts.28.3468

CHAPTER 17
COMMON SHOULDER DYSFUNCTIONS

By the end of this chapter you will understand:

- Anatomy
- Scapular dyskinesis
- Pathologies
  - o Acromioclavicular sprain
  - o Impingement
  - o Instability
  - o Subacromial bursitis
- Treatment options
  - o Early intervention
  - o Exercise intervention
    - Mobility/stability
    - Movement
    - What to avoid

Shoulder Anatomy

In simple terms, the shoulder joint is a shallow socket housing a small ball. The shoulder complex has three bones; the clavicle, the scapula, and the humerus (Oatis, 2017). This triaxle design allows for three degrees of freedom, and eight movements; flexion, extension, abduction, adduction, horizontal flexion, horizontal extension, internal rotation, and external rotation. The clavicle supports the upper extremity and is attached to the axioskeleton. The clavicle provides a base for muscle attachment, helps transmit force, and offers a base for shoulder stability while allowing for a range of motion (ROM) of 360 degrees. The scapula is primarily a stabilizer, but also allows for some mobility, and the proximal head of the humerus provides attachments for the four muscles of the rotator cuff (Oatis, 2019). The entire shoulder complex has four joints as detailed in Table 17.1 and Figure 17.1.

Table 17.1

Articulations of the shoulder

Joint	Articulation
Sternoclavicular	Between the manubrium of the sternum and the clavicle bone
Scapulothoracic	Between the scapula and the thorax
Acromioclavicular	Between the clavicle and scapula
Glenohumeral	Between the humeral head and the glenoid fossa of the scapula.

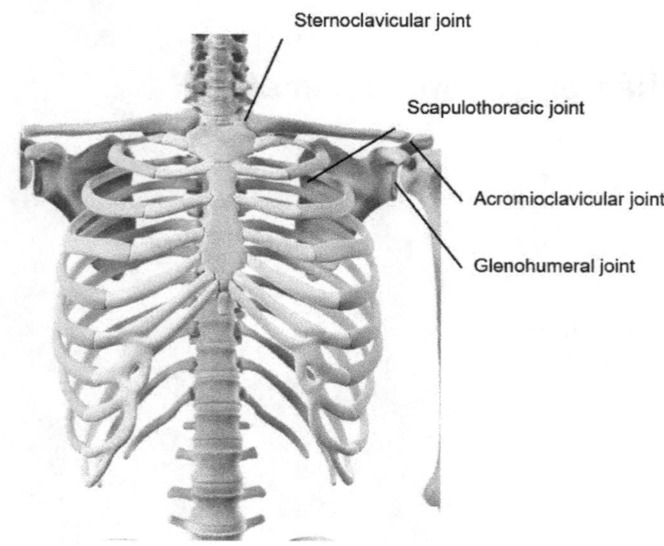

Figure 17.1 The joints of the shoulder (Shoulderdoc, 2019).

The sternoclavicular joint is formed by the medial end of the clavicle and the upper portion of the sternum, and provides 30-35 degrees of upward elevation, up to 35 degrees forward and backward movement, and 45-50 degrees of rotation (Terry & Chopp, 2000). Seventeen muscles attach to, or originate from the scapula which allows the scapulothoracic joint to provide mobility and stability to the glenohumeral (GH) joint via translation and rotation that includes (Oatis, 2017; Terry & Chopp, 2000):

- Elevation and depression
- Abduction and adduction
- Medial and lateral rotation
- Internal and external rotation
- Anterior and posterior tilt

The GH is the ball (humeral head) and socket (glenoid fossa) joint most commonly referred to as the shoulder joint, and is the most mobile joint in the human body allowing for flexion and extension, abduction and adduction, and internal and external rotation (Oatis, 2017). Mobility of the GH is controlled by supporting structures including the labrum, ligaments, and four rotator cuff muscles. The labrum is a thin rim of cartilage located around the edge of the glenoid socket that extends the socket by 5-9 mm. A damaged labrum can decrease shoulder mobility by as much as 20%, and strength by as much as 10%.

The rotator cuff is four small muscles that assist with dynamic stabilization of the glenohumeral joint: the subscapularis (not shown), the supraspinatus, the infraspinatus, and the teres minor as shown in Figure 17.2.

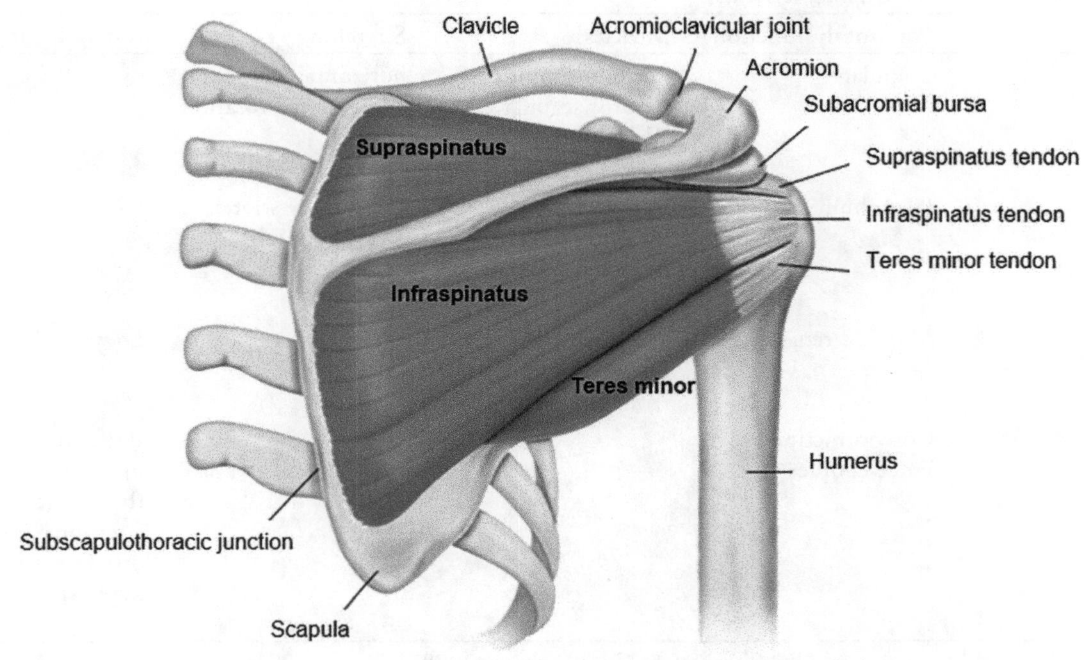

Figure 17.2 Rotator cuff and shoulder impingement

Scapular Dyskinesis

In Chapter four, Postural and Movement Assessments and Corrective Strategies, it was explained the scapula is primarily used for stabilization. Muscles that assist with dynamic stabilization of the GH joint originate from the scapula, and the scapula coordinates movement with the humerus to ensure efficient arm movements (Cools et al., 2014; Kibler et al., 2013). Scapular dyskinesis (SD) refers to altered or dysfunctional movement patterns, or the loss of normal control of the scapula (Kibler et al., 2013). Traumatic injury, neurological impairment, or muscular imbalance can cause SD. SD is characterized by scapula winging, shrugging or elevation, medial boarder prominence, or rounded shoulders. Although the exact causal relationship is unknown, SD is associated with many shoulder injuries including labral tears, rotator cuff injuries, AC separation, and multidirectional shoulder instability (Cools et al., 2014; Kibler et al., 2013; Levinson, 2015).

Altered movement patterns associated with SD can be the result of soft-tissue inflexibility and/or poor muscular performance. Overactive pectoralis minor can cause scapular and glenohumeral internal rotation and anterior tilting, similar to dysfunction associated with impingement syndrome, and chronic pain associated with overhead movements. Additionally, overactive levator scapulae, latissimus dorsi, external rotators, and rhomboids have been associated with restricted ROM of the scapula (Cools et al., 2014). Underactive muscles and muscles associated with poor scapular coordination include serratus anterior and all three sections of the trapezius, often resulting in increased shoulder elevation or shrugging during activation, and neck pain. See Table 17.2 for exercise recommendations for SD.

Table 17.2

Exercise recommendations for scapular dyskinesis

Concern	Point of dysfunction	Muscles	Stretching	Strengthening
Overactive	Scapular	Pectoralis minor Levator scapula Rhomboids	horizontal abduction and external rotation (Ts)	
	Glenohumeral	Posterior capsule Infraspinatus Latissimus Dorsi	Cross body stretch Sleeper stretch	
Underactive	Muscle strength	Serratus anterior Lower/middle traps		Low row Lawnmower Robbery
Coordination	Co-contraction Force couples			Posterior tilt and upward rotation of the thoracic spine (sternum up, head up, decrease thoracic kyphosis)

Cools et al., 2014; Kibler, Sciascia, Uhl, Tambay, & Cunningham, 2008; Levinson, 2015

Shoulder Pathologies

Shoulder separation

The acromioclavicular (AC) joint is located at the lateral border of the clavicle and the medial edge of the acromion. Due to the position and the small area of the AC joint, axial loading, such as weightlifting, heavy labor, or athletic activities can lead to joint problems, including osteoarthritis (Terry & Chopp, 2000). However, the most common mechanism for AC, or shoulder separation, are activities that often result in falling on an outstretched shoulder (Levinson, 2015; Li et al., 2014; Oatis, 2017). Most AC joint injuries are partial separation or sprains and are classified as Type I-VI as detailed in Table 17.3. Types IV-VI almost always require surgical intervention; Types I and II, and in some cases type III, may be managed without surgery.

Table 17.3

AC joint Injury and sprain classifications

Type	Characterizations	Managed without surgery
I	Stretched ligaments; no tear	Yes
II & III	Ligament tears with some deformity of the joint	Type II yes Type III varies
IV-VI	Complete tears of the AC ligaments; separation and damage to the surrounding structures	Almost never

Levinson, 2015; Li et al., 2014

Shoulder impingement

Shoulder impingement, often referred to as rotator cuff tendonitis or rotator cuff disease, has various pathologies (Ellenbecker & Cools, 2010; Escamilla, Hooks, & Wilk, 2014; Levinson, 2015). Primary impingement can occur when the supraspinatus tendon, the subacromial bursa, and the long biceps tendon (not shown) pass under coracoacromial arch (the ligament connecting the acromion and the coracoid process of the scapula [not shown]) placing the tissue at risk during shoulder flexion (Figure 17.2). Pain caused by impingement is progressive, often starting with bursitis, followed by partial to complete tears of the supraspinatus tendon, followed by damage to surrounding tissue. Impingement can also occur when the humeral head moves forward causing impingement of the supraspinatus and infraspinatus on the posterosuperior edge of the glenoid rim, leading to rotator cuff tears and labrum damage. Regardless of the mechanism of injury, shoulder impingement is usually associated with overuse, poor body mechanics, capsule laxity, and overhead motions like those performed when swimming, throwing, or in racquet sports (Ellenbecker & Cools, 2010; Escamilla, et al., 2014; Levinson, 2015). The likelihood of rotator cuff disease can also increase with age, obesity, and diabetes (Greenberg, 2014).

Subacromial bursitis

Subacromial bursitis is most often thought of as an overuse injury and can lead to rotator cuff tendonitis and impingement (Levinson, 2015). Subacromial bursitis occurs when the bursa, which sits beneath the acromion and the superior surface of the supraspinatus (Figure 17.2), and the surrounding tissue are inflamed. The inflamed tendons can rub on adjacent bone, causing tears of varying size and degree, some of which, if left unattended may require surgical intervention.

Shoulder instability

Because the AC joint is the most mobile joint in the human body, it is susceptible to anterior and posterior instability. Anterior shoulder instability can be caused by a traumatic injury, overuse, and repetitive overhead movements such as throwing a ball or swinging a racquet. Posterior shoulder instability can be caused by overzealous pushing movements and exercises such as a heavy bench press or push-ups (Levinson, 2015).

Interventions

The goal of early intervention, or phase one, is to reduce pain and inflammation, and is usually achieved by period of immobilization. Phase one also includes restoring ROM and stability, preventing or reducing muscle atrophy, and restoring proprioception (Ma et al., 2014). Accordingly, given the known association between SD and other shoulder conditins, it is not surprising restorative exercise intervention begins with scapular stability and rotator cuff strengthening, coupled with core strength and kinetic chain coordination. Movements to avoid during the initial phase of recovery for anterior instability are abduction, external rotation, and extension. Movements in the frontal plane and are encouraged; T's and Ys for example, will provide resistance, while placing little stress on the joint capsule. Movements that stress the posterior of the joint capsule, such as push-ups and bench pressing should be avoided for individuals with posterior shoulder instability, as should internal rotation with shoulder extension, as often seen in the empty-the-can exercise, as this movement may increase the chance of impingement.

Beginning stability and mobility exercises for anterior shoulder instability should consist of exercises such as planking on a stability ball, wall push-ups, and quadrupeds, as isometrics and closed chain movements will encourage stability and promote proprioception. Clients with posterior shoulder instability can perform external and internal rotation (with a band), serratus punches, or light, wide-grip bench press. Movement training can use isotonic push-ups, rowing, shoulder extension, and shrugs. Stability and mobility training for rotator cuff injuries, such as impingement, include the scapula strengthening movements used for shoulder instability, but should also include stabilization and strengthening exercises for the core, abdomen, and low back to improve proximal stability and posture. Internal and external rotation can be incorporated as inflammation is reduced. See Table 17.4 for recommended exercises for clients with shoulder instability and rotator cuff injuries.

Table 17.4

Recommended exercises for shoulder sprain and instability, and rotator cuff injuries

Dysfunction	Early intervention	Stability/Mobility	Movement	Avoid
Shoulder Sprain	Surgery Immobilization for pain control Cryotherapy Isometrics: • Abduction • Flexion • Extension • Internal and external rotation	Strengthen: • Rotator cuff • Deltoids • Pectoralis • Trapezius • Rhomboids • Latissimus Dorsi Begin with bands or very light weights and progress as needed	Functional movements to challenge the core and shoulders	Horizontal abduction and adduction Extreme scapular retraction or protraction Overhead or incline activities
Anterior Instability	A short period of immobilization Decrease pain and inflammation Restore ROM	Restore scapular stability Isometric and closed kinetic chain Plank on ball Wall push ups Quadruped—hold and stabilize Scapular dip	With scapular stability restored incorporate open kinetic chain Rowing Shrugs Serratus punch	Abduction External rotation Extension Behind the neck exercises

Posterior Instability	A short period of immobilization Decrease pain and inflammation Restore ROM	Internal rotation External rotation	Rowing External rotation Extension Horizontal abduction	Movements that push the humeral head posteriorly into the shoulder joint such as a bench press
Shoulder Impingement	Reduce inflammation Restore neuromuscular coordination	Restore scapular stability Rowing Push-ups with scapular protraction Shrugs Serratus punch Internal rotation External rotation Incorporate low back and core exercises to progress	Shoulder flexion T-Y Flexion Abduction External rotation	Overhead activities Overhead press Incline press Lateral raises Empty the can

Cools et al., 2014; Levinson, 2015

Discussion and application

1. Describe the importance of the scapula in restorative exercises for the shoulder and provide some examples of exercises that may improve shoulder dysfunctions.

References

Cools, A. M., Struyf, F., De Mey, K., Maenhout, A., Castelein, B., & Cagnie, B. (2014). Rehabilitation of scapular dyskinesis: From the office worker to the elite overhead athlete. *British Journal of Sports Medicine, 48*(8), 692-697. https://doi.org/10.1136/bjsports-2013-092148

Ellenbecker, T. S., & Cools, A. (2010). Rehabilitation of shoulder impingement syndrome and rotator cuff injuries: An evidence-based review. *British Journal of Sports Medicine, 44*(5), 319-327. https://doi.org/10.1136/bjsm.2009.058875

Escamilla, R. F., Hooks, T. R., & Wilk, K. E. (2014). Optimal management of shoulder impingement syndrome. *Open Access J Sports Med, 5*, 13-24. https://doi.org/10.2147/OAJSM.S36646

Greenberg, D. L. (2014). Evaluation and treatment of shoulder pain. *Medical Clinics of North America, 98*(3), 487-504. https://doi.org/10.1016/j.mcna.2014.01.016

Kibler, W. B., Sciascia, A. D., Uhl, T. L., Tambay, N., & Cunningham, T. (2008). Electromyographic analysis of specific exercises for scapular control in early phases of shoulder rehabilitation. *American Journal of Sports Medicine, 36*(9), 1789-1798. https://doi.org/10.1177/0363546508316281

Kibler, W. B., Ludewig, P. M., McClure, P. W., Michener, L. A., Bak, K., & Sciascia, A. D. (2013). Clinical implications of scapular dyskinesis in shoulder injury: The 2013 consensus statement from the 'Scapular Summit'. *British Journal of Sports Medicine, 47*(14), 877-885. https://doi.org/10.1136/bjsports-2013-092425

Levinson, M. (2015). Musculoskeletal injuries of the upper extremity in J.S. Skinner, C.X. Bryant, S. Merrill, & D.J. Green (Eds), *American Council on Exercise medical exercise specialist manual.* San Diego, CA: American Council on Exercise.

Li, X., Ma, R., Bedi, A., Dines, D. M., Altchek, D. W., & Dines, J. S. (2014). Management of acromioclavicular joint injuries. *The Journal of Bone & Joint Surgery, 96*(1), 73-84. https://doi.org/10.2106/JBJS.L.00734

Ma, R., Brimmo, O. A., Li, X., & Colbert, L. (2017). Current concepts in rehabilitation for traumatic anterior shoulder instability. *Current Reviews in Musculoskeletal Medicine, 10*(4), 499-506. https://doi.org/10.1007/s12178-017-9449-9

Oatis, C. (2017). *Kinesiology: The mechanics and pathomechanics of human movement* (3rd ed.). Philadelphia, PA: Wolters Kluwer.

Shoulderdoc. (2019). Four joints of the shoulder [jpeg image]. Retrieved from https://www.shoulderdoc.co.uk/article/1177

Terry, G. C., & Chopp, T. M. (2000). Functional anatomy of the shoulder. *Journal of Athletic Training, 35(*3), 248-255. Retrieved from http://natajournals.org/loi/attr

CHAPTER 18
COMMON DYSFUNCTIONS OF THE DISTAL ARM

By the end of this chapter you will understand:

- Anatomy
- Pathologies
    - o Epicondylitis
    - o Carpal Tunnel Syndrome
    - o De Quervain's Tenosynovitis
- Treatment options
    - o Early intervention
    - o Exercise intervention
        - ▪ Mobility/stability
        - ▪ Movement
        - ▪ What to avoid

Anatomy

The elbow is a hinge joint where the distal end of the humerus connects to the proximal ends of the ulna and radius. The elbow has two degrees of freedom; flexion and extension, and allows rotation, or pronation and supination of the forearm and wrist. The distal end of the humerus has two bony prominences called *epicondyles*. The proximal end of the ulna connects to the medial epicondyle and the proximal end of the radius connects at the lateral epicondyle as shown in Figure 18.1. Because many of the muscles that cross the elbow connect to the shoulder or wrist, a dysfunction at one joint can often result in a dysfunction at the next proximal or distal joint.

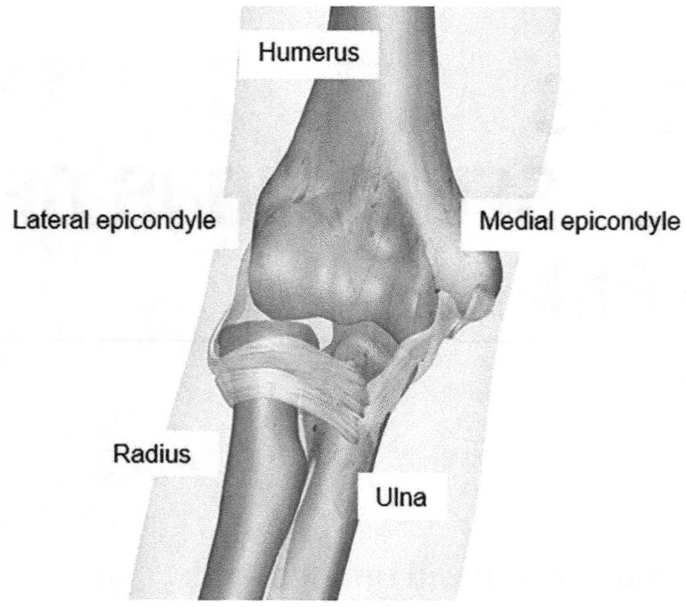

Figure 18.1 Elbow anatomy

Epicondylitis

Two common injuries to the elbow are lateral and medial epicondylitis, or tennis elbow and golfer's elbow that occur due to poor mechanics during activities with large force at the elbow joint. It is thought lateral epicondylitis results from the overuse of the wrist and forearm extensors and supinator muscles; however, the exact underlying cause is often difficult to discern (Ahmed et al., 2013). Often associated with tennis, other activities such as typing or playing a piano, carrying heavy weights, or repetitive elbow extension can also lead to lateral epicondylitis. Medial epicondylitis is often the result of repetitive eccentric loading during wrist flexion and forearm extension coupled with elbow valgus and pronation during activities such as golfing, overhead throwing, and swimming (Amin, Kumar, & Schickendantz, 2015). Both medial and lateral epicondylitis have historically been thought of as inflammatory responses, or tendonitis, the first phase of injury. However, repeated stress creates micro tears of the tendons resulting in tendinosis, a degenerative process characterized by structural breakdown and irreparable fibrosis or calcification (Ahmed et al., 2013; Amin et al., 2015).

The first line of treatment is to eliminate the movements that cause pain. When movements can be performed with little discomfort, the next step is to restore a pain free range of motion (ROM), followed by stability and mobility, and then movement. Similar to shoulder dysfunction, the elbow and wrist can also be affected by scapular dyskinesis. Therefore, it is prudent to assess the scapula and correct any dysfunctions as shown in Table 17.3. Please see Table 18.1 for specific guidelines for restorative exercises for epicondylitis.

Carpal Tunnel Syndrome

Carpal tunnel syndrome (CTS) results from the compression of the medial nerve in the carpal tunnel. The carpal tunnel is on the palmer side of the wrist. The floor and sides are made up of small carpal bones and cartilage, and the top is the transverse carpal, or palmar ligament (Figure 18.2). High-load, manual tasks, and repetitive pinching and finger tapping activities can create pressure in the carpal tunnel, causing swelling and edema (Ballestero-Perez; 2017; Levinson, 2015; Oatis, 2017). The median nerve is one of three major nerves that innervate the forearm and hand (Figure 18.2). Entrapment of the median nerve in the carpal tunnel due to swelling can cause tingling, pain, numbness, and weakness in the hand and fingers (Oatis, 2017). Additionally, CTS is often bilateral as the swelling can be caused by obesity, diabetes, arthritis, or hypothyroidism (Burton, Chesterton, & Davenport, 2014).

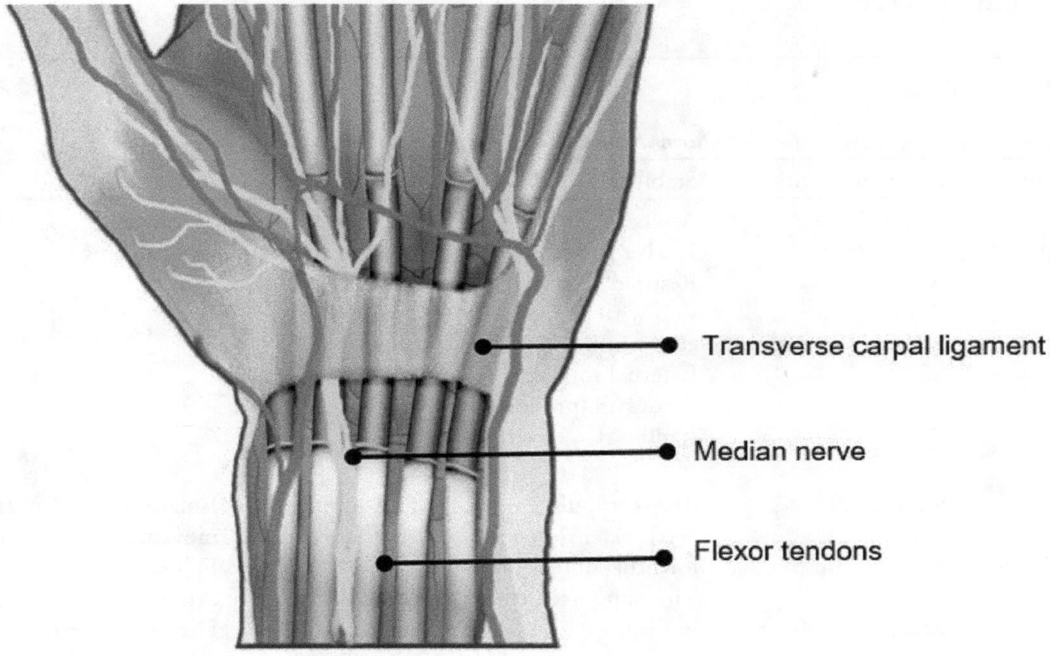

Figure 18.2 Carpal tunnel

On the ultraconservative end, CTS may resolve on its own in 12-15 months with splinting and avoiding aggravating activities. On the more aggressive end, surgery to release the transverse carpal ligament may be needed if conservative treatments fail. Non-steroidal anti-inflammatories (NSIADS), splints, and corticoid steroid injections are considered the most effective intervention for CTS. Regardless, restorative exercise should be part of a comprehensive treatment plan.

The goal of a restorative exercise program is to improve ROM while reducing pain. Although the research is limited, nerve and tendon gliding have been shown to be effective for mobilization, it is suggested they be incorporated during later stages of therapy or avoided altogether due to potential stretching of the median nerve (Ballestero-Perez; 2017; Carlson et al., 2010; Levinson, 2015). All other exercise treatments should begin with isometrics, followed by isotonic, eccentric, and then concentric (Levinson, 2015). See Table 18.1 for specific guidelines.

De Quervain's Tenosynovitis

De Quervain's tenosynovitis or De Quervain's disease is characterized by pain at the base of the thumb at the first dorsal compartment (Howell, 2012; Levinson, 2015; Rabin, Israeli, & Kozol, 2015). Tenosynovitis is the inflammation of the fluid-filled sheath (the *synovium*) that surrounds a tendon, typically leading to joint pain, swelling, and stiffness. Considered an overuse injury, movements requiring tight gripping such as golf and fishing, or repetitive tapping such as texting and typing, as well as other activities where the hand twists and bends, such as knitting, can cause tissue micro-trauma that result in the thickening of the extensor retinaculum of the wrist, leading to pain and swelling. Finkelstein's test, when the thumb and ulnar are tightly grasped and the hand is quickly deviated resulting in sharp pain, is the best way to differentiate De Quervain's tenosynovitis from other conditions (Howell, 2012). The treatment protocol for De Quervain's tenosynovitis is similar to CTS and can begin once the inflammation is controlled. Table 18.1 indicates specifics.

Table 18.1

Recommended restorative exercises for distal arm dysfunction

Dysfunction	Early intervention	Stability/Mobility	Movement	Avoid	Sets/Reps
Lateral Epicondylitis	Stop painful movements Restore pain free ROM Restore coordination	Assess scapula Passive wrist flexion Resisted wrist extension with supported elbow in flexion External rotation Ts and Ys (prone and standing)	Multi-joint exercises that replicate ADLs Rows Shrugs Lat pull downs	Strenuous weightlifting	Low resistance, high reps. 3 sets 15-20 reps
Medial Epicondylitis	Stop painful movements Restore pain free ROM Restore coordination	Assess scapula Wrist extension and forearm supination with supported elbow in flexion	Multi-joint exercises that replicate ADLs Stabilization, pushing, and pulling movements	Isolation movements Full elbow extension Heavy bicep curls	Low resistance, high reps. 3 sets 15-20 reps
Carpel Tunnel	NSAIDS Corticosteroids Splinting Reduce aggravating activities	Wrist extension/ flexion Radial and ulnar deviation Forearm pronation/ supination Finger flexion/ extension	Yoga Gripping exercises	Until pain subsides: Wrist flexion and extension >30 degrees Radial and ulnar deviation	

De Quervain's Tenosynovitis	NSAIDS Corticosteroids Splinting Reduce aggravating activities	Wrist extension/ flexion Radial and ulnar deviation Forearm pronation/ supination Finger flexion/ extension	Gripping exercises	Until pain subsides: Wrist flexion and extension >30 degrees Radial and ulnar deviation

Ahmed, et al., 2013; Amin et al., 2015; Ballestero-Perez; 2017; Carlson et al., 2010; Howell, 2012; Levinson, 2015; Rabin, Israeli, & Kozol, 2015

Discussion and application

1. What are some of the causes of epicondylitis and describe the major focus of restorative exercises and the rationale behind it.

References

Ahmad, Z., Siddiqui, N., Malik, S. S., Abdus-Samee, M., Tytherleigh-Strong, G., & Rushton, N. (2013). Lateral epicondylitis: A review of pathology and management. *The Bone and Joint Journal, 95-B*(9), 1158-1164. https://doi.org/10.1302/0301-620X.95B9.29285

Amin, N. H., Kumar, N. S., & Schickendantz, M. S. (2015). Medial epicondylitis: Evaluation and management. *Journal of the American Academy of Orthopaedic Surgeons, 23*, 348-355. https://doi.org/10.5435/JAAOS-D-14-00145

Ballestero-Perez, R., Plaza-Manzano, G., Urraca-Gesto, A., Romo-Romo, F., Atin-Arratibel, M. L., Pecos-Martin, D.,...Romero-Franco, N. (2017). Effectiveness of nerve gliding exercises on carpal tunnel syndrome: A systematic review. *Journal of Manipulative & Physiological Therapeutics, 40*(1), 50-59. https://doi.org/10.1016/j.jmpt.2016.10.004

Burton, C., Chesterton, L. S., & Davenport, G. (2014). Diagnosing and managing carpal tunnel syndrome in primary care. *The British Journal of General Practice, 64*(622), 262-263. https://doi.org/10.3399/bjgp14X679903

Carlson, H., Colbert, A., Frydl, J., Arnall, E., Elliot, M., & Carlson, N. (2010). Current options for nonsurgical management of carpal tunnel syndrome. *International Journal of Clinical Rheumatology, 5*(1), 129-142. https://doi.org/10.2217/IJR.09.63

Howell, E. R. (2012). Conservative care of De Quervain's tenosynovitis/ tendinopathy in a warehouse worker and recreational cyclist: A case report. *The Journal of the Canadian Chiropractic Association, 56*(2), 121-127. Retrieved from https://www.chiropractic.ca/jcca-online/issue/june-2012-volume-56-2/

Levinson, M. (2015). Musculoskeletal injuries of the upper extremity in J.S. Skinner, C.X. Bryant, S. Merrill, & D.J. Green (Eds), American Council on Exercise medical exercise specialist manual. San Diego, CA: American Council on Exercise

Oatis, C. (2017). *Kinesiology: The mechanics and pathomechanics of human movement* (3rd ed.). Philadelphia, PA: Wolters Kluwer

Rabin, A., Israeli, T., & Kozol, Z. (2015). Physiotherapy management of people diagnosed with de Quervain's Disease: A case series. *Physiotherapy Canada, 67*(3), 263-267. https://doi.org/10.3138/ptc.2014-47

CHAPTER 19
COMMON HIP DYSFUNCTIONS

By the end of this chapter you will understand:

- Anatomy
- Pathologies
    - o Gluteal Trochanteric Pain Syndrome and Trochanter Bursitis
    - o IT band friction syndrome
    - o Osteoarthritis
    - o Hip replacement
    - o Piriformis syndrome
- Treatment options
    - o Early intervention
    - o Exercise intervention
        - ▪ Mobility/stability
        - ▪ Movement
        - ▪ What to avoid

Anatomy

Similar to the shoulder, the hip is a ball and socket joint with three degrees of freedom that allows movement in all planes of motion. The hip joint is formed from the proximal head of the femur and the pelvic acetabulum. Also similar to the shoulder, the acetabulum has a ring of fibrous cartilage, the *acetabular labrum*, which adds depth to the hip socket and provides stability for weight bearing movements. Figure 19.1 diagrams the hip socket, and Table 19.1 details the movements of the hip and its involved muscles.

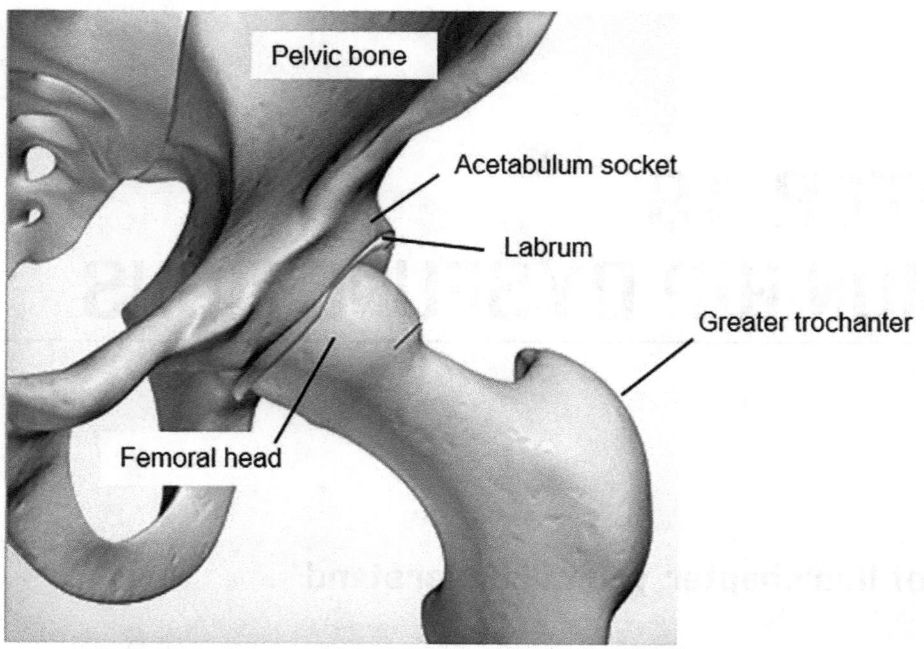

Figure 19.1 Diagram of the hip

Table 19.1

Movements of the hip and the involved muscles

Movement	Involved Muscles
Flexion	iliopsoas, rectus femoris, sartorius, pectineus
Extension	gluteus maximus and hamstrings: semimembranosus, semitendinosus, and biceps femoris
Abduction	gluteus medius, gluteus minimus, piriformis and tensor fascia latae
Adduction	adductors longus, brevis and magnus, pectineus and gracilis
Lateral rotation	biceps femoris, gluteus maximus, piriformis, assisted by the obturators, gemilli and quadratus femoris
Medial rotation	anterior fibers of gluteus medius and minimus, tensor fascia latae

(Cheatham, 2015; Mallow & Nazarian, 2014):

Gluteal Trochanteric Pain Syndrome and Trochanter Bursitis

Common hip conditions are trochanteric pain syndrome, iliotibial (IT) band friction syndrome (ITBFS), and arthritis that may lead to hip replacement. The trochanters are two bony protuberances toward the top of the femur and serve as sites for muscle attachment. The greater trochanter is at the junction of the neck and shaft of the femur. The muscles that insert on, or near the greater trochanter are the gluteus medius and minimus, piriformis, obturator externus, and obturator internus. Greater trochanteric pain syndrome (GTPS) refers to hip pain such as bursitis and tendonitis (Cheatham, 2015; Mallow & Nazarian, 2014).

Trochanteric bursa are located on the lateral side of the greater trochanter and provide protection for the gluteus medius and minimus, the IT band, and the tensor fascia lata (TFL). Trochanteric bursitis is inflammation of the bursa between the greater trochanter and the gluteus medius and IT complex. Inflammation can be caused by age, an accident or trauma, repetitive movements such as running or kicking, as well as structural and muscular dysfunctions. Trochanteric bursitis can often result in low back pain, pain radiating down the lateral aspect of the thigh to the knee, pain when walking, and pain when lying on the effected side. Reduced strength and range of motion have also been associated with trochanteric bursitis. It is now known that extreme cases of trochanter inflammation may be the result of tears in the gluteus minimus and medius; similar to rotator cuff tears that lead to tendinopathy (Cheatham, 2015; Mallow & Nazarian, 2014).

Due to the many reasons for hip pain, it is strongly recommended a client with hip pain get a clinical diagnosis prior to beginning an exercise program. Hip pain may be the result of:

- Gluteus medius dysfunction, gluteus medius or gluteus minimus tendinopathy
- Piriformis tendinopathy
- Iliotibial tract friction syndrome
- Trochanteric bursitis
- Piriformis syndrome
- Osteoarthrosis
- Acetabular labral tear
- Femoral neck fracture
- Iliopsoas tendinopathy
- Hernia
- Intervertebral disk disease
- Lumbosacral dysfunction or disease
- Lumbosacral spine sprain or strain
- Sacroiliac joint injury or dysfunction
- Referred pain from intra-abdominal processes

Iliotibial Band Friction Syndrome

The IT band is a thick portion of lateral fascia of the upper leg that crosses over the hip and knee joints and overlays the greater trochanter. It originates at the iliac crest and inserts at the lateral condyle of the tibia and helps with movement and stability in the lower extremity as shown in Figure 19.2 (Lavine, 2010; Hyland & Varacallo, 2018). Because of the anatomical structuring of the IT band, it is presumed Iliotibial band friction syndrome (ITBFS) is an overuse injury caused by repetitive tightening of lateral fascia resulting in a compressive force to IT band connective tissue.

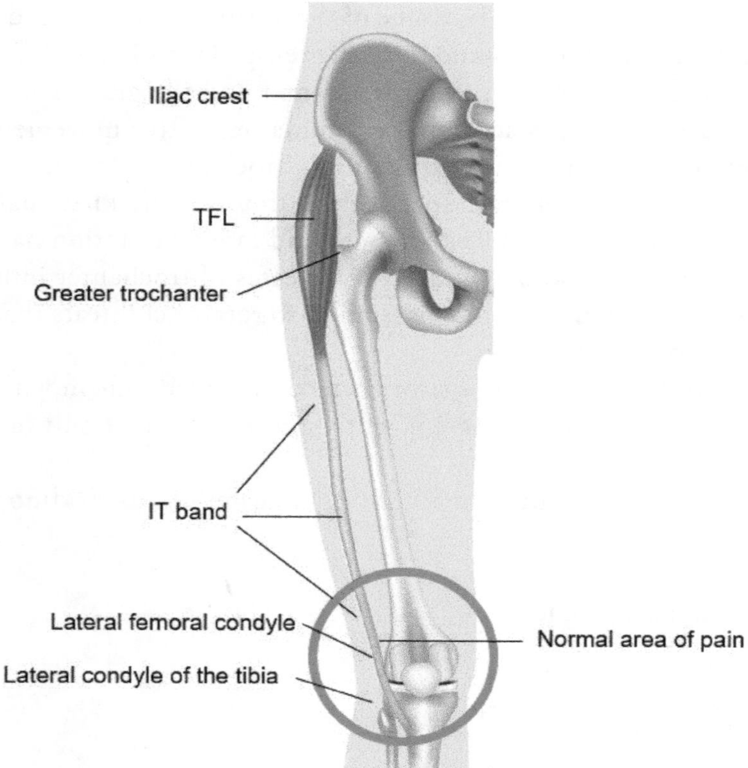

Figure 19.2 IT band syndrome.

ITBFS is the most common knee injury reported in runners, but also common in cyclists. Because ITBFS often manifests as pain originating from the lateral femoral condyle (figure 19.2), it was originally thought to be an overuse injury related to repetitive movement of the knee; however, it is now thought ITBFS could be caused by repetitive movement of the hip, its actual pathology is unknown (Cheatham, 2015; Lavine, 2010). What is known are heavy landing forces, increased knee internal rotation, and quadriceps that are comparatively stronger or more active than the same side hamstrings are biomechanical factors associated with ITBFS. Pain or tenderness may be gradual, starting at the knee and working up the lateral aspect of the thigh, and there may also be a snapping or popping at the knee during extension and flexion. Restorative exercise recommendations for GTPS and ITBFS are in Table 19.3.

Osteoarthritis

Osteoarthritis (OA) is a degenerative disease that develops when the cartilage and supporting joint structures deteriorate. It is estimated over 31 million American adults suffer from OA, with age as the single most determining factor. Although it is thought everyone over the age of 60 suffers from OA in at least one joint, it is known 70% of people over the age of 65 suffer from OA (Cibulka et al., 2009). Additionally, OA is more prevalent in people who suffer from other chronic disease (Arthritis Foundation, n.d.):

- 49% of adults with heart disease have arthritis
- 47% of adults with diabetes have arthritis
- 31% of adults who are obese have arthritis

OA effects an entire joint from increased tensile loads on the joint capsule, and compressive forces on the remaining cartilage. Obesity, genetic anomalies, leg length discrepancy, hip dysplasia, cysts, bone spurs, a limited range of motion (ROM), and muscle weakness are associated with hip OA. Weak core musculature, abductors, and gluteus medius can cause muscle imbalances and dysfunction and may lead to a Trendelenberg gait pattern, an abnormal gait characterized by a hip drop or trunk lean (Cibulka et al., 2009). A deep aching pain during weight bearing activities, joint stiffness in the morning or after a period of inactivity, and joint instability are classic signs of hip OA. These indications can also be attributed to other conditions such as bursitis, stress fracture, muscle or labral tears, piriformis syndrome, or sacroiliac joint dysfunction; therefore, it is imperative a client seeks medical permission prior to an exercise program. Due to deficits in proprioception, stability and balance training should be included in any restorative exercise program for a client with hip OA. A list of interventions for hip OA are in Table 19.3.

Hip Replacement

It is estimated more than 300,000 total hip replacements or total hip arthroplasty (THA) are performed each year in the United States on patients age 45 and older. There are approximately 2.5 million adults in the United States living with a total hip replacement (Maradit Kremers et al., 2015; Wolford, Palso, & Bercovitz, 2015). Although the most common cause for THA is OA, rheumatoid arthritis, bone fractures, or other neurological or muscular disorders are also reasons for replacement. The main goal of THA is to reduce pain and improve quality of life.

Primary THA involves removing the damaged femoral head and replacing it with a metal stem with a ball on the end that is inserted into the femur; a metal or plastic socket replaces the damaged acetabulum. In a partial hip replacement, the femur side is replaced, but not the hip socket. For younger patients, bone resurfacing or remodeling is often performed, allowing a patient a number of years before needing a THA. Clients who have comorbidities such as osteoporosis, joint ligament laxity, or an infection are usually not eligible for hip replacement surgery.

Primary hip replacement is usually performed using a posterior-lateral approach, an anterior-lateral approach, or a direct anterior approach (Chetham, 2015; Ritterman & Rubin, 2013). The posterior-lateral approach disrupts the external rotators (piriformis, gemelli, obturtators, quadratus femoris), while the anterior-lateral approach disrupts the gluteus minimus and medius, and the abductor muscles. The direct anterior approach is becoming popular as it spares all of the involved muscles and nerves. Each approach has restrictions, and movements and activities to avoid are listed in Table 19.3.

Piriformis Syndrome

Piriformis syndrome is pain of the hip or buttock that may radiate down the posterior thigh and lower leg (Tonely et al., 2010). The piriformis is a flat, triangular shaped muscle that sits deep to the gluteal muscles with its origin at the ilium and the 2nd and 4th sacral vertebrae, and insertion at the greater trochanter as seen in Figure 19.2 (Dey, Das, & Bhattacharyya, 2013; Hicks& Varacallo, 2018; Huber & Palmer, 2018). The piriformis is mostly used for external rotation at the hip, but assists in hip flexion, abduction, and internal rotation when the hip is flexed to 90 degrees (Boyajian-O'Neill, McClain, Coleman, & Thomas, 2008; Huber & Palmer, 2018).

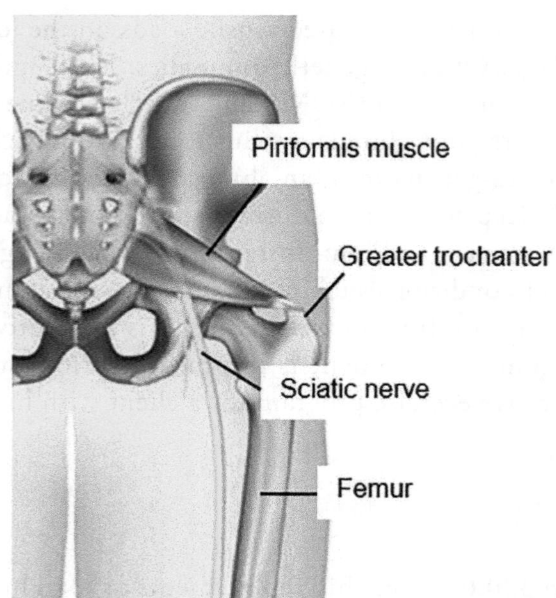

Figure 19.3 Diagram of the piriformis muscle

In most people, the sciatic nerve runs inferior to the piriformis muscle; however, in 12-22% of the population, the sciatic nerve runs through, or splits, the piriformis. Pain from this anatomical arrangement is known as primary piriformis syndrome and is responsible for approximately 15% of diagnosed piriformis syndrome cases (Boyajian-O'Neil et al., 2008; Dey et al., 2013). Secondary piriformis syndrome is caused by macro-trauma to the buttocks or micro-trauma caused by repetitive movements such as running, or sitting on a hard surface (fat wallet syndrome), which leads to inflammation, and poor blood flow to the tissue. The inflamed piriformis muscles then compress the sciatic nerve against the pelvis. Piriformis syndrome is thought to be responsible for up to 6% of low back pain, discussed further in Chapter 22. Symptoms, contributing factors, and risk factors are detailed in Table 19.2.

Table 19.2

Symptoms, contributing factors, and risk factors for piriformis syndrome

Symptoms	Contributing factors	Risk factors
Pain with sitting, standing, or lying longer than 15 to 20 minutes	Excessive contraction of the piriformis muscle	Previous trauma
Radiating pain from sacrum through gluteal area and the posterior aspect of thigh	Weak or lengthened piriformis muscle	Sitting for long periods on hard surfaces
Pain improves with movement and worsens while sedentary	Spasm or repetitive contracture	Anatomical variations of the piriformis
Pain moving into an upright position	Trauma to buttocks or surrounding tissue which may have occurred several years previously	Leg length discrepancy,
Pain does not go away when position is changed	Inflammation	Lumbar hyperlordosis

Contralateral sacroiliac pain	Asymmetrical pelvis,	Repetitive physical activities
Difficulty walking	Core instability	Conditions that cause spasticity
Numbness in foot	Sacroiliac joint or pelvic malalignment	Total hip replacement
Weakness in same side lower extremity	Excessive localized pressure—mostly from sitting	Females are at higher risk due to Q-angle
Abdominal, pelvic, and inguinal pain	SI joint inflammation	Middle age
Pain with bowel movements	Myositis ossificans (bone in the muscle)	
Tenderness of muscle or surrounding tissue		
Limited medial rotation on same side		
Atrophy of the gluteal muscles		

Dey et al., 2013; Huber& Palmer, 2018

Early, conservative treatment relives symptoms in almost 80% of diagnosed cases (Boyajian-O'Neill et al., 2008; Dey et al., 2013). As with all hip injuries, a medical diagnosis should rule out conditions presenting with similar manifestations such as spinal stenosis, spondylolisthesis, disc herniation, pelvic fracture, or internal disorders such as endometriosis or renal stones (Huber & Palmer, 2018). Activities can resume when there is a pain-free range of motion with increased strength on the affected side (Hicks & Varacallo, 2018). Restorative exercise recommendations are detailed in Table 19.3.

Table 19.3

Restorative exercise recommendations for common hip injuries

Condition	Early intervention	Mobility/Stability	Movement	Avoid
Trochanteric bursitis and Iliotibial band friction syndrome	Physical therapy Anti-inflammatories Steroids Surgery	Static stretching, PNF, and myofascial release of the hamstrings and gluteus medius OKC exercises Side lying clams Adduction and abduction	Progressive functional exercises to improve ADLs, core, and balance Wall squats Leg press Multi-directional lunges Side steps Start in bi-lateral stance Followed by staggered and monoped while decreasing stability	Activities that aggravate the condition

Total hip arthroplasty				
Posterior-lateral	Improve strength Improve ROM Stretching and myofascial release Check with physician and physical therapist to determine appropriate course of action	Restore strength, proprioception, and neuromuscular control Stretching to mild or moderate discomfort Static PNF SMR	Focus on core, lumbo-pelvic-hip complex with functional movements Sit-to-stand Stairs Bending Balance progression	Hip flexion > 90 degrees Adduction past midline I/R past neutral High impact activities
Anterior-lateral		Focus on the glutes, IT band, hamstrings, and quads OKC strengthening with light weights or bands	Low-load, non-weight bearing cardiovascular conditioning appropriate for deconditioned client	E/R combined with flexion Adduction past midline I/R past neutral High impact activities
Direct anterior				Hyperextension E/R High impact activities
Piriformis syndrome	Ice Rest NSAIDs Steroid injections	Stretches that involve hip and knee flexion, hip adduction, and internal rotation Corrective exorcises to address faulty movement patterns Core stabilization exercises Bridges with abduction Clam shells	Hip adductor strengthening Squats with abduction Side steps (tube walks) Multi-planar lunges Functional movements to incorporate ADLs	Aggravating movements until there is a pain free ROM and unilateral strength

Aronen & Lorenz, 2015; Cheatham, 2015; Cibulka et al., 2009; Dey et al., 2013; Huber & Palmer, 2018; Lavine, 2010; Jogi, Overend, Spaulding, Zecevic, & Kramer, 2015; Mallow & Nazarian, 2014; Ritterman & Rubin, 2013; Tonely et al., 2010

Discussion and application

1. What is the difference between a sprain and a strain, how can these be avoided, and what is the protocol in dealing with a sprain or strain?
2. What are some common hip dysfunctions, and what are the goals for restorative exercise for each. Describe examples of exercises to consider and avoid.

References

Aronen, J. G., & Lorenz, K. A. (2015). Arthritis in J.S. Skinner, C.X. Bryant, S. Merrill, & D.J. Green (Eds), *American Council on Exercise medical exercise specialist manual.* San Diego, CA: American Council on Exercise.

Arthritis Foundation. (n.d.). Arthritis facts. Retrieved from https://www.arthritis.org/about-arthritis/understanding-arthritis/arthritis-statistics-facts.php.

Boyajian-O'Neill, L. A., McClain, R. L., Coleman, M. K., & Thomas, P. P. (2008). Diagnosis and management of piriformis syndrome: An osteopathic approach. *Journal of American Osteopathic Association, 108*(11), 657-664. Retrieved from https://jaoa.org/Issue.aspx#issueid=932088

Cheatham, S. (2015). Musculoskeletal injuries of the lower extremity in J.S. Skinner, C.X. Bryant, S. Merrill, & D.J. Green (Eds), *American Council on Exercise medical exercise specialist manual.* San Diego, CA: American Council on Exercise.

Cibulka, M. T., White, D. M., Woehrle, J., Harris-Hayes, M., Enseki, K., Fagerson, T. L.,…Godges, J. J. (2009). Hip pain and mobility deficits--hip osteoarthritis: Clinical practice guidelines linked to the international classification of functioning, disability, and health from the orthopaedic section of the American Physical Therapy Association. *Journal of Orthopaedic & Sports Physical Therapy 39*(4), A1-25. https://doi.org/10.2519/jospt.2009.0301

Dey, S., Das, S., & Bhattacharyya, P. (2013). Piriformis syndrome: A clinical review. *Journal of Evolution of Medical and Dental Sciences, 2(*15), 2502-2508. Retrieved from https://www.jemds.com

Hicks, B. L., & Varacallo, M. (2018). *Piriformis Syndrome.* StatPearls [Internet]. Treasure Island, FL: StatPearls Publishing.

Huber, L., & Palmer, E. (2018). *Clinical review: Piriformis syndrome.* Glendale, CA: Cinahl Information Systems.

Hyland, S., & Varacallo, M. (2018). *Anatomy, bony pelvis and lower limb, iliotibial band (tract*). Treasure Island, FL: StatPearls Publishing.

Jogi, P., Overend, T. J., Spaulding, S. J., Zecevic, A., & Kramer, J. F. (2015). Effectiveness of balance exercises in the acute post-operative phase following total hip and knee arthroplasty: A randomized clinical trial. *SAGE Open Med, 3,* 2050312115570769. https://doi.org/10.1177/2050312115570769

Lavine, R. (2010). Iliotibial band friction syndrome. *Current Reviews in Musculoskeletal Medicine, 3(*1-4), 18-22. https://doi.org/10.1007/s12178-010-9061-8

Maradit Kremers, H., Larson, D. R., Crowson, C. S., Kremers, W. K., Washington, R. E., Steiner, C. A.,…Berry, D. J. (2015). Prevalence of total hip and knee replacement in the United States. *The Journal of Bone and Joint Surgery, 97(*17), 1386–1397. https://doi.org/10.2106/JBJS.N.01141

Mallow, M., & Nazarian, L.N. (2014). Greater trochanteric pain syndrome diagnosis and treatment. *Physical Medicine and Rehabilitation Clinics of North America, 25*(2), 279-289. https://doi.org/10.1016/j.pmr.2014.01.009

Ritterman, S., & Rubin, L. E. (2013). Rehabilitation for total joint arthroplasty. *Rhode Island Medical Journal, 96*(5), 19-22. Retrieved from http://www.rimed.org/rimedicaljournal-about.asp

Wolford, M. L., Palso, K., & Bercovitz, A. (2015). Hospitalization for total hip replacement among inpatients aged 45 and over: United States, 2000-2010. NCHS Data Brief (186), 1-8

CHAPTER 20
COMMON KNEE DYSFUNCTIONS

By the end of this chapter you will understand:

- Anatomy
- Pathologies
  - o Patellofemoral pain syndrome
  - o Meniscus tear
  - o ACL rupture
  - o Knee replacement
- Treatment options
  - o Early intervention
  - o Exercise intervention
    - ▪ Mobility/stability
    - ▪ Movement
    - ▪ What to avoid

Anatomy

The knee is a complex hinge joint that allows for 6 degrees of freedom; 3 rotational, and 3 translational motions. The tibiofemoral joint is where the distal portion of the femur articulates with the proximal tibia. The patellofemoral joint is where the patella (kneecap) and femur meet. The knee joint has four main movements; flexion, extension, medial rotation, and lateral rotation, with lateral and medial rotation occurring only when the knee is flexed.

The knee has five main ligaments and two menisci. The menisci are c-shaped, fibrocartilage structures attached to the medial and lateral ends of the intercondylar area of the tibia (Figure 20.3). They help stabilize the knee by deepening the articular surface of the tibia, they increase surface area that dissipates shock and force, and because of the location of mechanoreceptors, help with proprioception (Fox, Bedi, & Rodeo, 2012). The ligaments are:

- Patellar ligament is the distal portion of the quadriceps femoris tendon that connects to the patella and the tibial tuberosity.
- Medial collateral ligament (tibial) attaches to the medial epicondyle of the femur and the medial condyle of the tibia.
- Lateral collateral (fibular) ligament attaches to the lateral epicondyle of the femur and on the lateral surface of the fibular head
- Posterior cruciate ligament (PCL) attaches at the posterior intercondylar of the tibia and anteromedial femoral condyle.
- Anterior cruciate ligament (ACL) attaches at the anterior intercondylar of the tibia and posteriorly on the medial surface of lateral condyle of the femur.

The collateral ligaments stabilize the hinge motion and prevent excessive medial and lateral rotation. The PCL prevents posterior dislocation of the tibia with the femur, and the ACL prevents anterior dislocation of the tibia with the femur. Figure 20.1 details knee anatomy.

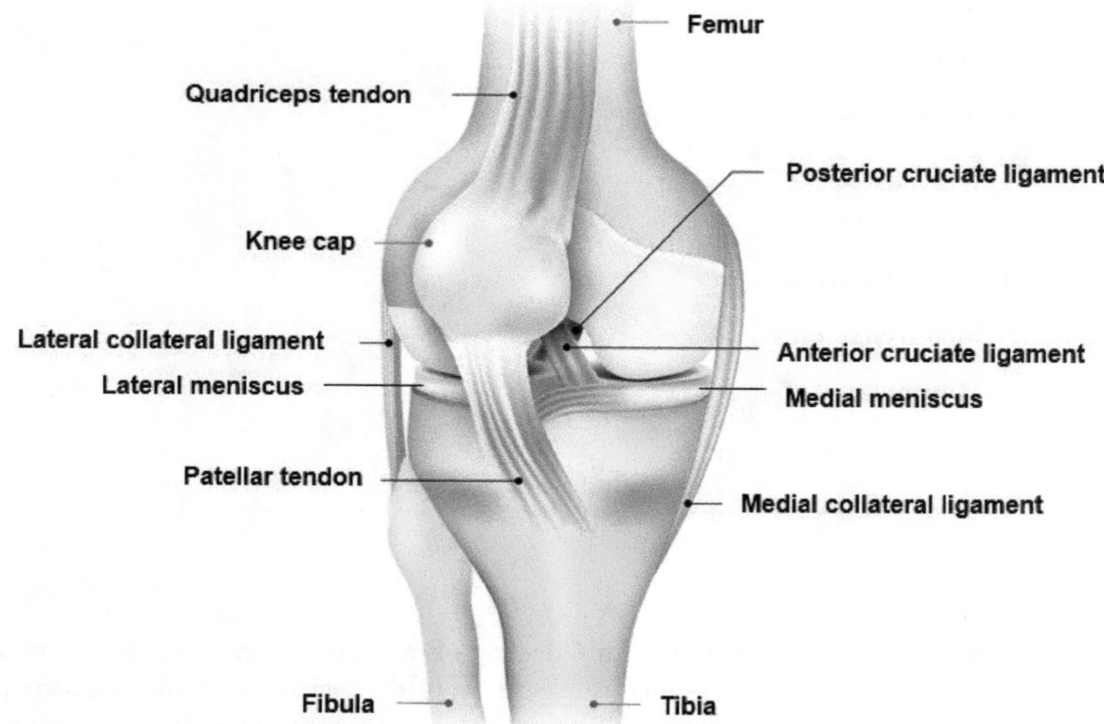

Figure 20.1 Diagram of front right knee

Patellofemoral Pain Syndrome

Patellofemoral pain syndrome (PFPS) is characterized by stiffness and pain during or following squatting, lunging, climbing or descending stairs, prolonged sitting, or running (Cheatham, 2015; Dixit, Difiori, Burton, & Mines, 2007). Popping, catching, or clicking sensations have also been associated with PFPS as the kneecap moves in and out of the trochlear groove. Swelling of the knee, instability, or locking **are not** characteristic of PFPS, and because PFPS is just one possible diagnosis for knee pain (some other possibilities are listed below), it is imperative a client presenting with knee pain consult a physician.

Possible causes for anterior knee pain:

- Tumor
- Iliotibial band syndrome
- Osgood-Schlatter disease
- Patellar bursitis
- Quadriceps or patellar tendinopathy
- Patellar instability/subluxation
- Chondromalacia patellae

Often referred to as *runner's knee* or anterior knee pain, PFPS is a common diagnosis for patients presenting with knee pain, and the most common diagnosis for runners (Bolgla & Boling, 2011; Dixit et al., 2007). Common risk factors for PFPS are overuse, trauma, muscle dysfunction (overactive and under active muscles), and structural or anatomical abnormalities. Sudden training program changes such as increased frequency or intensity can contribute to tissue damage, joint injury, and pain. Repetitive loading can lead to overuse injuries of the knee. Running, climbing stairs, hill ascending and descending, and jumping are all activities that can lead to PFPS.

Because the knee is the crossing point between the hip and ankle, over and underactive muscles from the hip, upper leg, and lower leg can cause abnormal movement patterns that disrupt normal knee function (Sahrmann, 2011). Due to the connection, via fascia, between the iliotibial (IT) band and the knee, an overactive IT band complex can pull the knee laterally. Therefore, flexibility in the IT band complex should be assessed. Underactive knee extensors and external hip rotators are associated with patella tracking dysfunction, knee valgus and excessive pronation suggests strengthening the entire quadriceps group, as well as the hip complex via extension and abduction may be beneficial. Keep in mind, although strengthening the quadriceps is the gold standard for restorative exercise for PFPS, the flexibility of hamstrings, hip flexors, and gastrocnemius should be assessed and treated to avoid excessive contact between the patella and femur because of increased posterior force. Restoring neuromuscular control of the hip complex should be part of the initial focus of restorative exercise (Bolgla & Boling, 2011; Cheatham, 2015; Dixet et al., 2007).

Q-angle

Although structural and anatomical abnormalities is out of the scope of practice for a CXS, it is important to know how biomechanical dysfunctions can affect movement patterns. The Q-angle is the measurement between the quadriceps muscles and the patella tendon. To determine the Q-angle, draw a line from the anterior superior iliac crest to the center of the kneecap, and another line from the center of the kneecap to the tibial tuberosity as shown in Figure 20.2. The Q-angle is important; it is thought to reflect of the effectiveness of the pull of the quadriceps on the patella: the greater the angle, the less effective the pull, as well as increased knee adduction and foot pronation. This has come under scrutiny as of late, and although it may be implicated in some knee conditions, it is important to remember the Q-angle cannot be changed. Therefore, a more effective approach is to correct the increased femoral and tibial internal rotation and femoral abduction (Bolgla & Boling, 2011). Flat feet and high arches (pes planus and pes cavus), have also been associated with PFPS. Clients with flat feet may compensate for a lack of foot stability by presenting with increased tibial and femoral internal rotation. Similarly, high arches cannot provide proper cushioning or reflexive mechanical energy assistance during loading activities such as jumping or running. In addition to restoring flexibility and strength, stability and mobility training should also focus on restoring neuromuscular control to the hips, knees, and ankles; movement training should focus on progressive functional exercises to improve ADLs. Suggestions for working with clients who have been diagnosed by a physician with PFPS are in Table 20.1.

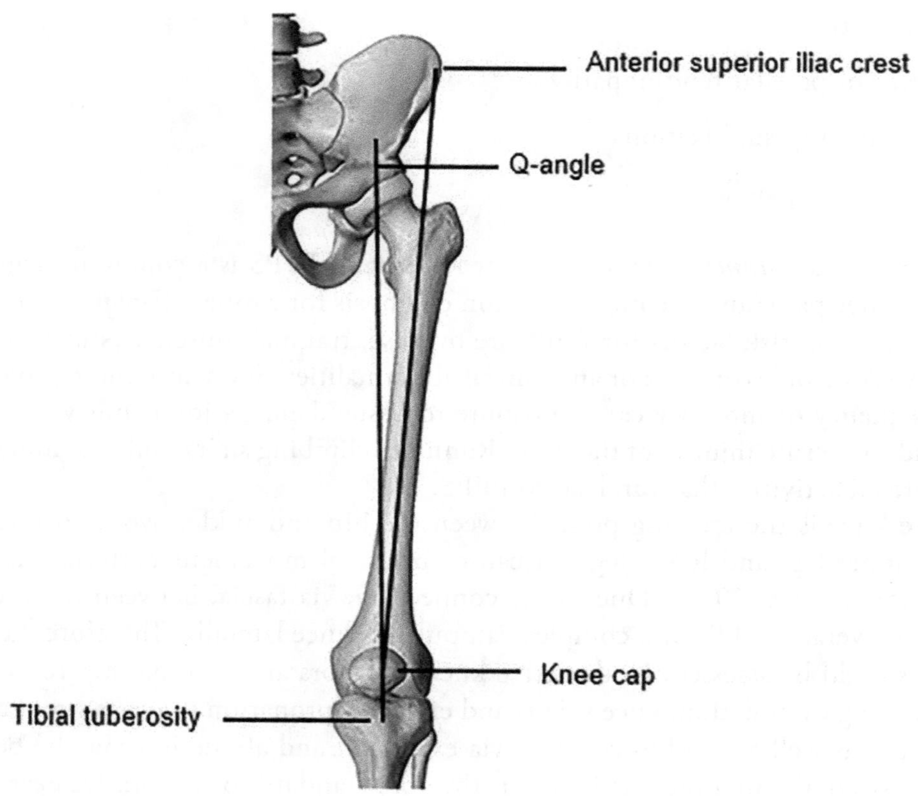

Figure 20.2 Diagram of the Q-angle.

Meniscus Injuries

Meniscus injuries can be either acute (traumatic) or chronic (degenerative), and occur when fibrocartilage tears or splits, usually due to axial loading and rotational force that create a shearing force across the tibiofemoral compartments of the knee (Doral, Bilge, Huri, Turhan, & Verdonk, 2018; Pekkerman, Ralhan, & Chang, 2017). It is important to remember menisci are part of a complex network of ligaments and bony attachments and should not be treated as separate structures. Furthermore, while at birth, each meniscus is vascularized, by adulthood, only 10-30% of the meniscus outer periphery, or red zone, has blood flow as diagramed in Figure 20.3.

Signs of a meniscus tear are knee pain, stiffness, clicking, popping, catching, locking, swelling, and muscle weakness (Cheatham, 2015). Risk factors for meniscal tears are age > 60, male, active work involving squatting, kneeling, or climbing stairs, the sports of soccer and rugby, and waiting >12 months after ACL injury and corrective surgery (Doral et al., 2018). Tears are generally described by location and type and include vertical longitudinal tears that can degenerate into a bucket handle, oblique, transverse or radial, horizontal tears that run parallel to the tibial plateau and can lead to a flap tear, meniscal root tear or avulsion that occur near the root insertion, and complex or degenerative tears that are a combination of tear patterns, as detailed in Figure 20.3. The most common traumatic tears are longitudinal-vertical and the most common site for tears is the posterior horn on the medial meniscus. Tears in the vascular zone often heal faster than tears in the avascular zone, and may heal spontaneously (Howell, Kumar, Patel, & Tom, 2014). The most common side effect resulting from a meniscal surgery is osteoarthritis.

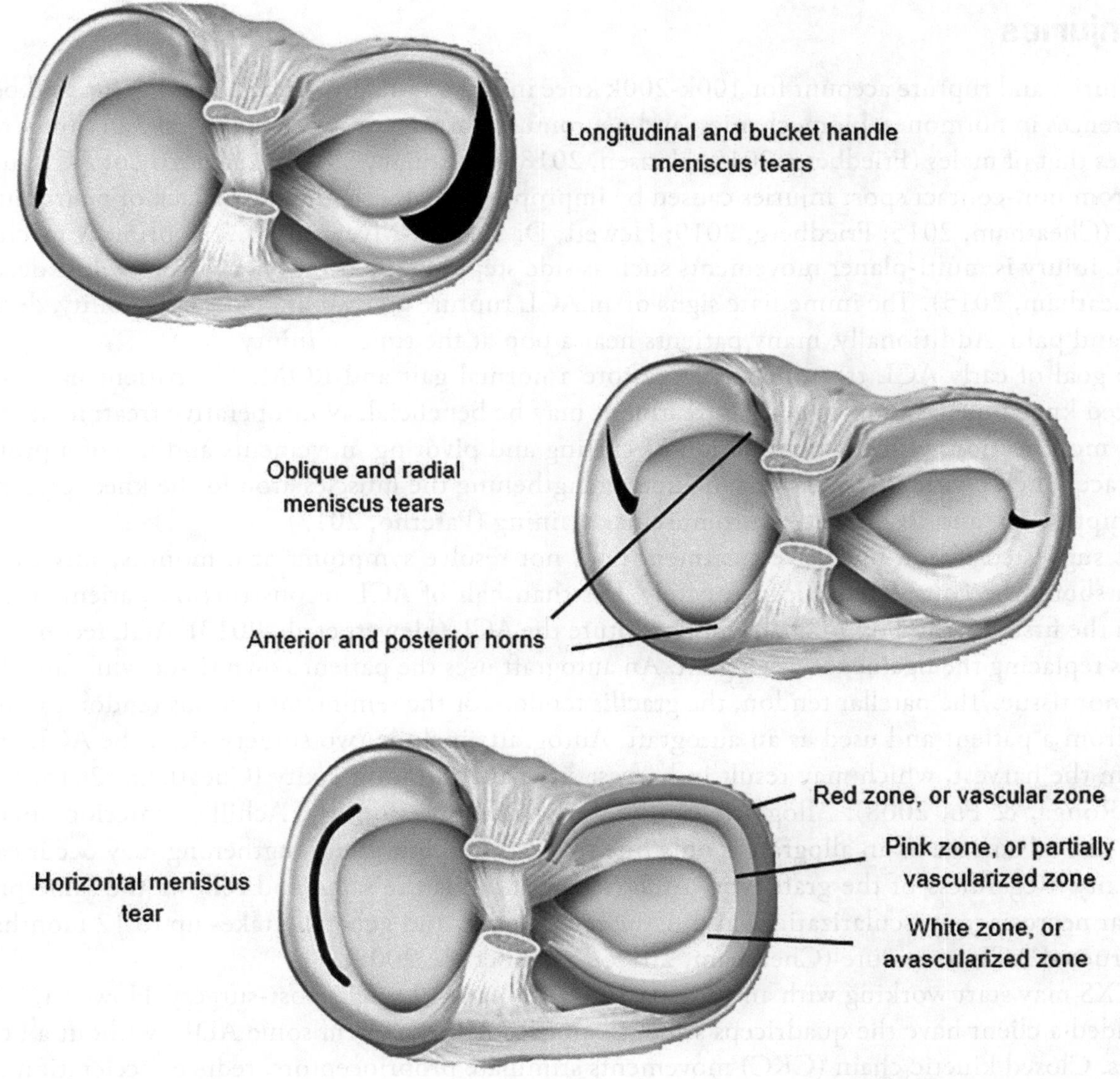

Figure 20.3 Diagrams of common meniscus tears and *vascularization*.

Immediately post-injury, protection, rest, ice, compression, and elevation are recommended with anti-inflammatory and analgesic medications. For the first 6 months activity modification with an unloader-brace is suggested as is quadriceps strengthening. If non-operative management fails to relieve symptoms, surgery should be considered (Cheatham, 2015; Doral et al., 2018; Howell et al., 2014). Surgery may involve partial or complete removal of the meniscus or suturing the torn fragment. Removal can lead to joint degeneration and repairs are most effective if a tear is in the vascular zone.

A CXS may work with a client who had a partial or complete meniscectomy 4 weeks post-surgery or a client who had a meniscus repair 12 weeks post-surgery. Early physical therapy intervention consists of quad sets, straight leg raises (SLR), heel raises, balance, and flexibility. Mid-phase rehab includes light leg press, step-ups, calf raises, and partial squats. Range of motion (ROM) should not be attempted until swelling is minimized and 110 degrees of flexion is reached. Late-phase rehab is dedicated to continuing the progress and achieving activities of daily living (ADLs). You must consult with a physical therapist and/or physician prior to starting a training program. Restorative protocols are in Table 20.1.

ACL Injuries

ACL injuries and rupture account for 100k-200k knee injuries annually in the United States and because of differences in hormones, biomechanics, and neuromuscular adaptation, females have an injury rate up 3.5 times that of males (Friedberg, 2019; Hansen, 2018; Voskanian, 2013). A majority of ACL ruptures result from non-contact sport injuries caused by improper body mechanics and a lack of neuromuscular control (Cheatham, 2015; Friedberg, 2019; Hewett, Di Stasi, & Myer, 2013). The primary mechanism for ACL injury is multi-planer movements such as side stepping, pivoting, or twisting, while decelerating (Cheatham, 2015). The immediate signs of an ACL rupture are swelling, knee instability, decreased ROM, and pain. Additionally, many patients hear a pop at the time of injury.

The goal of early ACL treatment is to restore a normal gait and ROM. If a patient has no other associated knee injuries, non-operative treatment may be beneficial. Non-operative treatments include activity modification with the elimination of cutting and pivoting movements and use of a protective knee brace. Therapeutic interventions include strengthening the muscles around the knee, cryotherapy and compression, and ROM and neuromuscular training (Paterno, 2017).

It is suggested if non-operative treatment does not resolve symptoms at 6 months, surgical intervention should be considered. Unfortunately, less than half of ACL reconstruction patients return to sport in the first year, and up to 25% will re-rupture the ACL (Hewett et al., 2013). ACL reconstruction involves replacing the ligament with a graft. An autograft uses the patient's own tissue while an allograft uses donor tissue. The patellar tendon, the gracilis tendon, or the semimembranosus tendon can be harvested from a patient and used as an autograft. Autografts include two surgery sites, the ACL and the site from the harvest, which may result in harvest site pain and joint laxity (Cheatham, 2015; Ekdahl, Wang, Ronga, & Fu, 2008). Allografts can be donor tendons from the Achilles, anterior tibialis, or patella. The advantage of an allograft is only one surgical site, but graft lengthening may occur causing joint laxity. Regardless of the graft type, ACL healing time is the same and follows the same process; avascular necrosis, re-vascularization, and tissue remodeling, and generally takes up to 12 months for a reconstructed ACL to mature (Cheatham, 2015; Ekdahl et al., 2008).

A CXS may start working with an ACL patient as soon as 12 weeks post-surgery. However, it is recommended a client have the quadriceps strength and ROM to perform some ADLs without a brace or crutches. Closed kinetic chain (CKC) movements stimulate proprioceptors, reduce acceleration forces, and encourage joint stability, while open kinetic chain (OKC) movements increase shear force across the knee joint. Therefore, it is recommended to start with CKC and progress to OKC, while keeping CKC movements to <90 degrees of flexion. Protocols for exercise training are in Table 20.1.

Total Knee Replacement

The incidence of total knee replacement, or arthroplasty (TKA), has increased over the last decade, with an estimated 4.5 million Americans living with TKA, and the incidence increase is expected to continue (Mayo Clinic, 2019). If one of the three components of the knee (femoral, tibial, or patellar), is damaged or arthritic, and physiotherapy or medical treatments such as anti-inflammatories, pain relievers, or bracing or assistive devises do not resolve symptoms a TKA, or a partial replacement may be necessary. During TKA all three components are replaced with plastic or metal; in a partial knee replacement, only one component is replaced. A TKA is preferred over a partial replacement because the components last longer and if two or more of the compartments are damaged, a TKA will need to be performed anyway (Cheatham, 2015).

There are no specific precautions or standardized rehabilitation guidelines, but it is recommended exercises should focus on reducing swelling, improving ROM, increasing knee and hip strength and proprioception, and restoring ADLs (Cheatham, 2015 Mistry et al., 2016). Particular focus should be given to the quadriceps as diminished muscle activation and weakness are known deficits following TKA. Additionally, because of surgery and motor control dysfunction, the quadriceps, hamstrings, and calves often become tight, so stretching the lower extremities is a common focus of restorative exercise post-TKA. Cardiovascular exercise should begin at a basic level and progress slowly. Aquatic exercise is a good place to start as it provides a non-weight bearing, buoyant medium to alleviate joint stress (Mistry et al., 2016). Exercise activity can begin at 6-12 weeks, and a CXS should consult a client's physician and physical therapist for specific guidelines. General restorative exercise guidelines are in Table 20.1. For a detailed list of rehabilitation guidelines, see Appendix 2 in Mistry et al. (2016).

Table 20.1

General activity guidelines for common knee dysfunctions

Condition	Early intervention	Stability/mobility	Movement	Avoid
PFPS	Modify activities to avoid pain Get fitted for footwear Braces, supports, orthotics Taping Anti-inflammatories	IT Band stretching and SMR Posterior chain stretching OKC quad movements: Straight leg raises Terminal knee extensions Leg extension between 90-60 degrees CKC movements for functional activity as tolerated Partial squat Side steps Step ups	Progressive functional exercises to improve ADLs, core, and balance. Wall squats Leg press Multi-directional lunges Side steps Start in bi-lateral stance Followed by staggered and monoped while decreasing stability Cardiovascular exercise should include low-loading exercises such as water aerobics and bicycle	Prolonged sitting with knees flexed Running Jumping Squats CKC movements between 30-60 degrees OKC movements between 25-0 degrees

Meniscus injury	Intervention following surgery depends on the type of surgery. Removal allows for a more aggressive approach than a repair. Bracing and non-weight bearing OKC exercises with some restrictions on ROM. Flexion to 90 degrees Extension to 30 degrees Light leg press to 10 degrees of ext.	Continue progress made in physical therapy Improve stretching for muscles that cross the knee: Hamstrings Quadriceps Neuromuscular training—balance progression	CKC movements start at <45 degrees and progress to 90 degrees; Leg press Squats Lunges Abduction/Adduction Leg ext. 90-60 degrees	Deep squats Pivoting Cutting Leg flexion past 90 degrees (lunges, leg press, etc.) Knee hyper extension Plyometrics
Knee replacement surgery	Physical therapy for 6-12 weeks Reduce swelling Increase knee and hip strength Improve balance and proprioception Begin restoration of ADLs	Flexibility throughout the hips, thighs, and claves pain free with a controlled ROM Gait training Neuromuscular training—balance progression SLR Quad sets	Low-load OKC exercises, SLR, and extension and flexion between 90-60 degrees CKC exercises from 0-45 degrees to start and progressing to 90 degrees Leg, press Wall squats, Multi-planer lunges,	High intensity movements until a base of strength and control has been established. Jumping Running Skiing Racquet sports Contact sports

Cheatham, 2015; Mistry et al., 2016; Saka, 2014; Stensrud, Roos, & Risberg, 2012

Discussion and application

1. What are the causes and signs of patellofemoral pain syndrome? What are the goals of a restorative exercise program, and what are some contraindications?
2. Describe the first few weeks of rehabilitation following meniscus surgery. At what point is it appropriate to begin working with a fitness professional as opposed to a physical therapist?

References

Bolgla, L. A., & Boling, M. C. (2011). An update for the conservative management of patellofemoral pain syndrome: A systematic review of the literature from 2000 to 2010. *International Journal of Sports Physical Therapy, 6*(2), 112-125. Retrieved from https://www.ncbi.nlm.nih.gov/pmc/articles/PMC3109895/

Cheatham, S. (2015). Musculoskeletal injuries of the lower extremity in J.S. Skinner, C.X. Bryant, S. Merrill, & D.J. Green (Eds), *American Council on Exercise medical exercise specialist manual.* San Diego, CA: American Council on Exercise.

Dixit, S., Difiori, J. P., Burton, M., & Mines, B. (2007). Management of patellofemoral pain syndrome. *American Family Physician, 75*(2), 195-202. Retrieved from http://www.aafp.org/afp/2007/0115/p194.html

Doral, M. N., Bilge, O., Huri, G., Turhan, E., & Verdonk, R. (2018). Modern treatment of meniscal tears. *EFORT Open Rev, 3*(5), 260-268. https://doi.org/10.1302/2058-5241.3.170067

Ekdahl, M., Wang, J. H., Ronga, M., & Fu, F. H. (2008). Graft healing in anterior cruciate ligament reconstruction. *Knee Surgery, Sports Traumatology, Arthroscopy, 16*(10), 935-947. https://doi.org/10.1007/s00167-008-0584-0

Fox, A. J., Bedi, A., & Rodeo, S. A. (2012). The basic science of human knee menisci: Structure, composition, and function. *Sports Health, 4*(4), 340-351. https://doi.org/10.1177/1941738111429419

Friedberg, R. (2019). Anterior cruciate ligament injury. In K.B. Fileds (Ed.). *UptoDate*. Retrieved April 13, 2020, from https://www.uptodate.com/contents/anterior-cruciate-ligament-injury

Hansen, M. (2018). Female hormones: Do they influence muscle and tendon protein metabolism? *Proceedings of the Nutrition Society, 77(*1), 32-41. https://doi.org/10.1017/S0029665117001951

Hewett, T. E., Di Stasi, S. L., & Myer, G. D. (2013). Current concepts for injury prevention in athletes after anterior cruciate ligament reconstruction. *American Journal of Sports Medicine, 41*(1), 216-224. https://doi.org/10.1177/0363546512459638

Howell, R., Kumar, N. S., Patel, N., & Tom, J. (2014). Degenerative meniscus: Pathogenesis, diagnosis, and treatment options. *World Journal of Orthopedics, 5*(5), 597-602. https://doi.org/10.5312/wjo.v5.i5.597

Mayo Clinic. (2019). Medical professionals: Orthopedic surgery. Retrieved from https://www.mayoclinic.org/medical-professionals/orthopedic-surgery/news/first-nationwide-prevalence-study-of-hip-and-knee-arthroplasty-shows-7-2-million-americans-living-with-implants/mac-20431170

Mistry, J. B., Elmallah, R. D., Bhave, A., Chughtai, M., Cherian, J. J., McGinn, T.,...Mont, M. A. (2016). Rehabilitative guidelines after total knee arthroplasty: A review. *The Journal of Knee Surgery, 29(*3), 201-217. https://doi.org/10.1055/s-0036-1579670

Paterno, M. V. (2017). Non-operative care of the patient with an ACL-deficient knee. *Current Reviews in Musculoskeletal Medicine, 10*(3), 322-327. https://doi.org/10.1007/s12178-017-9431-6

Pekkerman, B., Ralhan, P., & Chang, R. (2017). PM&R knowledge now: Meniscus injuries of the knee. *American Academy of Physical Medicine and Rehabilitation.* Retrieved from https://now.aapmr.org/

Sahrmann, S. (2011). *Movement system impairment syndromes of the extremities, cervical, and thoracic spines*. Atlanta, GA: Elsevier.

Saka, T. (2014). Principles of postoperative anterior cruciate ligament rehabilitation. *World Journal of Orthopedics, 5*(4), 450-459. https://doi.org/10.5312/wjo.v5.i4.450

Stensrud, S., Roos, E. M., & Risberg, M. A. (2012). A 12-Week exercise therapy program in middle-aged patients with degenerative meniscus tears: A case series with 1-year follow-up. *Journal of Orthopaedic & Sports Physical Therapy, 42*(11), 919-931. https://doi.org/10.2519/jospt.2012.4165

Voskanian N. (2013). ACL Injury prevention in female athletes: Review of the literature and practical considerations in implementing an ACL prevention program. *Current Reviews in Musculoskeletal Medicine, 6*(2), 158–163. https://doi.org/10.1007/s12178-013-9158-y

CHAPTER 21
COMMON DYSFUNCTIONS OF THE LOWER EXTREMITY

By the end of this chapter you will understand:

- Anatomy
- Pathologies
    - o Shin splints
    - o Ankle sprains
    - o Achilles Tendinopathy
    - o Plantar Fasciitis
- Treatment options
    - o Early intervention
    - o Exercise intervention
        - Mobility/stability
        - Movement
        - Precasutions

Anatomy

The lower extremity, the shin, ankle, and foot, is an essential structure for mobility and stability, and for any weight bearing activity. The shin is divided into four compartments: anterior, lateral, superficial posterior, and deep posterior. Table 21.1 lists the muscles of each compartment, and the associated movements, and Figure 21.1 provides a cross-sectional view of the lower extremity compartments.

Table 21.1

Compartments and muscles of the lower leg, and their actions

Compartment	Muscles	Actions
Anterior	Anterior tibialis Extensor digitorum longus Extensor hallucis longus Peroneus tertius	Dorsiflexion Inversion Toe extension Eversion and abduction—Peroneus tertius
Lateral	Peroneus longus Peroneus brevis	Plantarflexion Eversion
Superficial posterior compartment	Gastrocnemius Soleus Plantaris	Plantarflexion Knee flexion—Plantaris
Deep posterior compartment	Tibialis posterior Flexor digitorum longus Flexor hallucus longus Popliteus	Inversion Adduction Plantarflexion Supination Toe flexion Internally rotates tibia—Popliteus Assists with knee flexion—Popliteus

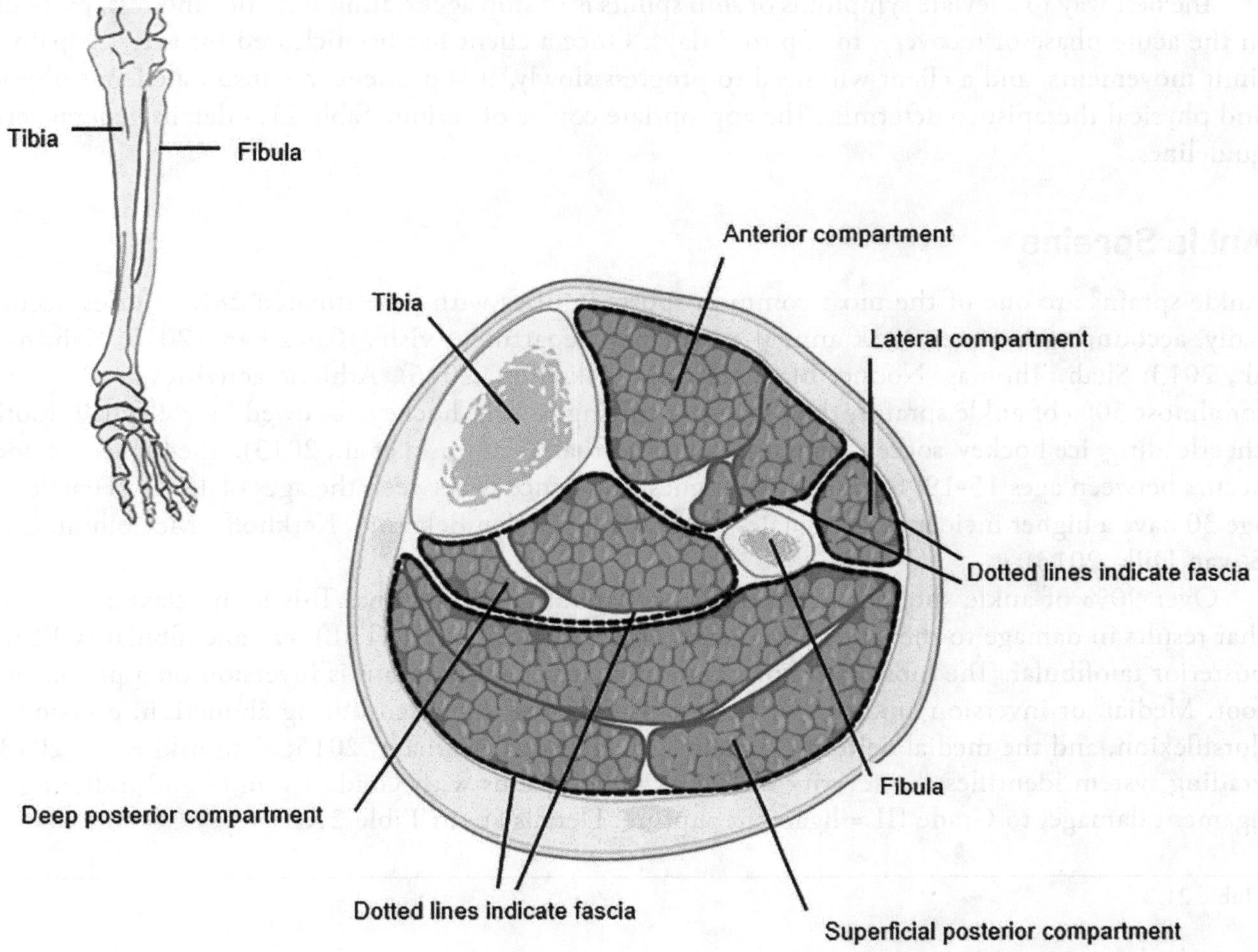

Figure 21.1 Diagram of the shin bones and a cross sectional view of lower extremity

Shin Splints

Shin splint is a generic term used to describe anterior or posterior lower leg pain. Posterior shin splints are also known as *medial tibial stress syndrome* (MTSS). The main cause of MTSS is inflammation of the periosteum, a layer of connective tissue that surrounds bone, or periostitis. However, in addition to periostitis, a range of tibial stress injuries that include tendinopathy and periosteal remodeling can also be a cause, as can dysfunction of the shin musculature (Galbraith & Lavallee, 2009). Anterior shin splints refer to pain in the muscles and fascia of the anterior compartment.

Shin splints are the result of repetitive muscle contraction and tibial strain caused by repetitive loading such as running, structural anomalies such as pes planus, leg length discrepancy, knee valgus or varus, muscular imbalances such as over active calf muscles, or poor biomechanics such as over pronation (Cheatham, 2015; Galbraith & Lavallee, 2009; Mandom & Paul, 2015). Shin splint pain is characterized by a dull ache or diffuse pain along the lower part of the medial tibia for MTSS, or lower anterior shin and compartment for anterior shin splints (Cheatham, 2015; Galbraith & Lavallee, 2009). Pain is often severe at the beginning of an exercise bout and diminishes as the bout continues, but as the condition progresses, the pain becomes continuous.

The best way to alleviate symptoms of shin splints is to stop aggravating activities and rest, particularly in the acute phase of recovery, for up to 7 days. Once a client has been cleared for activity, pain may limit movements, and a client will need to progress slowly. It is prudent to consult a client's physician and physical therapist to determine the appropriate course of action. Table 21.4 details general activity guidelines.

Ankle Sprains

Ankle sprains are one of the most common sports injuries with an estimated 28K injuries occurring daily, accounting for over 225k annual emergency department visits (Cheatham, 2015; Kaminski et al., 2013; Shah, Thomas, Noone, Blanchette, & Wikstrom, 2016). Athletic activities are responsible for almost 50% of ankle sprains, the highest occurring in field hockey, followed by volleyball, football, cheerleading, ice hockey, soccer, gymnastics, and softball (Kaminski et al., 2013). The highest incidence occurs between ages 15-19; for males the highest incidence is between the ages of 15-24. Females after age 30 have a higher incidence than males (Ott, 2013; van den Bekerom, Kerkhoffs, McCollum, Calder, & van Dijk, 2013).

Over 90% of ankle sprains are inversion, or lateral, ankle sprains. This is the classic *rolled ankle* that results in damage to the lateral ligaments, anterior talofibular (ATFL), calcaneofibular (CFL), and posterior talofibular. The most common cause of a lateral ankle sprain is inversion on a plantar flexed foot. Medial, or inversion ankle sprains occur when force is applied during abduction, eversion, and dorsiflexion, and the medial deltoid ligament is damaged (Cheatham, 2015; Kaminski et al., 2013). A grading system identifies the severity of lateral ankle sprains with Grade I = mild and indicting little ligament damage, to Grade III = ligament rupture. Details are in Table 21.2

Table 21.2

Lateral ankle sprain grading system

	Grade I	Grade II	Grade III
Ligaments involved	ATFL	ATFL & CFL	One or more
Ligament damage	Stretched	Stretched	Ruptured
Swelling/Tenderness	Mild	Moderate	Severe
Laxity/Stability	None-little	Abnormal	Substantial

American Academy of Orthopaedic Surgeons, 2019; Cheatham, 2015; Kaminski et al., 2013; Ott, 2013

A sprain heals in three phases and treatment should be adjusted as healing progresses. During Phase I, the initial or inflammatory phase, the RICE protocol (rest, ice, compression, and elevation) is the widely accepted intervention to reduce swelling and induce healing. RICE should be considered for 5-7 days, and the affected ankle should be kept immobile. Phase II is the proliferation phase that can last up to 3 months. During this stage, vascularity increases in the damaged tissue and new collagen forms. Controlled stress is encouraged to align the newly-formed tissue, but inversion should be avoided. Bracing, taping, and wrapping can keep the ankle stable. In Phase III, remodeling takes place, and activity becomes important. The newly-formed collagen is laid as scar tissue, and as this tissue develops, it is vital to stretch the ankle to breakdown scar tissue and align the fibers. The remodeling phase can take up to a year or longer (van den Bekerom et al., 2013).

A CXS can work with a client with a Grade I sprain as early as Week 1; Week 3 for a Grade II sprain, and Week 6 for a grade III sprain. Progressive weight bearing and functional rehabilitative activities may be a better than complete immobilization for Grades I or II sprains. Due to joint laxity and inhibited proprioception, the primary risk factor for an ankle sprain is a previous sprain. Therefore, it makes sense the best means of prevention and recovery is stability, balance, and neuromuscular training. Wobble boards, BOSUs, foam and air pads, and single leg movements should be performed. As always, check with a client's physician or physical therapist for progression protocol. Guidelines for activity are in Table 21.4.

Achilles Tendinopathy

The rate of incidence of Achilles tendon (AT) injuries is unknown, but ranges between 7–49/100,000, and affects an estimated 1 million athletes annually (Lemme, Li, DeFroda, Kleiner, & Owens, 2018; Shamrock & Varacallo, 2019). AT injuries mostly occur in intermittent athletes (weekend warriors), and most commonly affect middle-aged males. There are numerous intrinsic and extrinsic factors that can lead to AT injury and include:

- Age
- Bodyweight
- Pes planus and pes cavus
- Leg length discrepancy
- Limited calf flexibility
- Ankle instability
- Kidney disease
- Gout
- Diabetes
- Thyroid disorders
- Arthritis
- Infection
- Knee and hip dysfunction (Cheatham, 2015; Lemme et al., 2018; Shamrock & Varacallo, 2019)

Historically, AT pain has been associated with inflammation; however, it is now thought AT pain is more often a result of tendon degeneration, suggesting a more appropriate name may be *Achilles tendinosis*, or the more encompassing term of *Achilles tendinopathy* that indicate pain, swelling, degeneration, and dysfunction (Cheatham, 2015; Sussmilch-Leitch, Collins, Bialocerkowski, Warden, & Crossley, 2012). Symptoms often occur at the mid-line or distal portion of the of the tendon insertion with the calcaneus (Figure 21.2). The associated pain is present in the morning and as the severity of the condition increases, the sharp or burning pain occurs more often. Rest will usually alleviate the symptoms and should be considered as part of any recovery, but conservative physical therapy is the most widely accepted treatment (Sussmilch-Leitch et al., 2012).

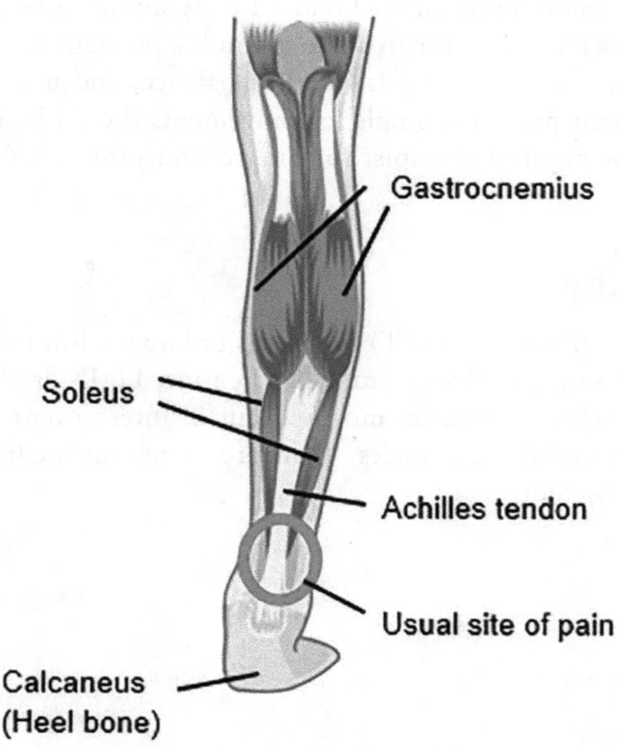

Figure 21.2 Achilles tendonitis.

Early intervention includes rest, oral or injectable anti-inflammatories, modification of risk factors, weight-loss, assessment of footwear or the addition of orthotics, assessment of body mechanics, and physical therapy with a focus on stretching and eccentric strengthening. High-intensity and high-loading activities should be avoided, and restrictions in the type and amount of activity may be necessary. Guidelines for activity are listed in table 21.4.

Plantar Fasciitis

The plantar fascia is a thick band of fibrous tissue that runs from the heel across the arch of the foot and connects to the ball of the foot (Figure 21.3). As the foot flattens, the plantar fascia acts as a shock absorber, or rubber band, and helps return the foot to its original arch (Kirby, 2017). Plantar fasciitis (PF) occurs when the fascia becomes strained or weakened, causing tears, swelling, and pain. More recently, the term *plantar fasciosis* is now used to indicate degeneration and disorganization of fibrous tissue rather than just inflammation. Some of the causes of PF are in Table 21.3.

Table 21.3

Plantar fasciitis risk factors

Intrinsic risk factors	Pes planus
	Pes cavus
	Obesity
	Shortened Achilles tendon
	Increased subtalar pronation
	Age
	Sex
	Overactive calf muscles
	Limited dorsiflexion
Extrinsic risk factors	Walking, standing, or running for long periods of time, especially on hard surfaces
	Improper foot wear
	Walking barefoot
	Sports or physical activity
	Overtraining
	Deconditioning
	Lack of flexibility training

(Bolivar, Munuera, & Padillo, 2013; Memorial Sloan Kettering Cancer Center, 2019; Schwartz & Su, 2014).

Approximately 2 million patients are treated for PF in the United States every year. The most commonly reported symptom of PF is pain in the medial heel at the calcaneal attachment as shown in Figure 21.3. Clients report pain particularly upon rising in the morning and taking a few steps. The pain can be severe at first but may subside after a few minutes of activity. The condition seems to worsen at night, due to increased plantar flexion and an overactive triceps surae (gastrocnemius and soleus) while sleeping (Bolivar et al., 2013). The pain often returns after prolonged standing or activity.

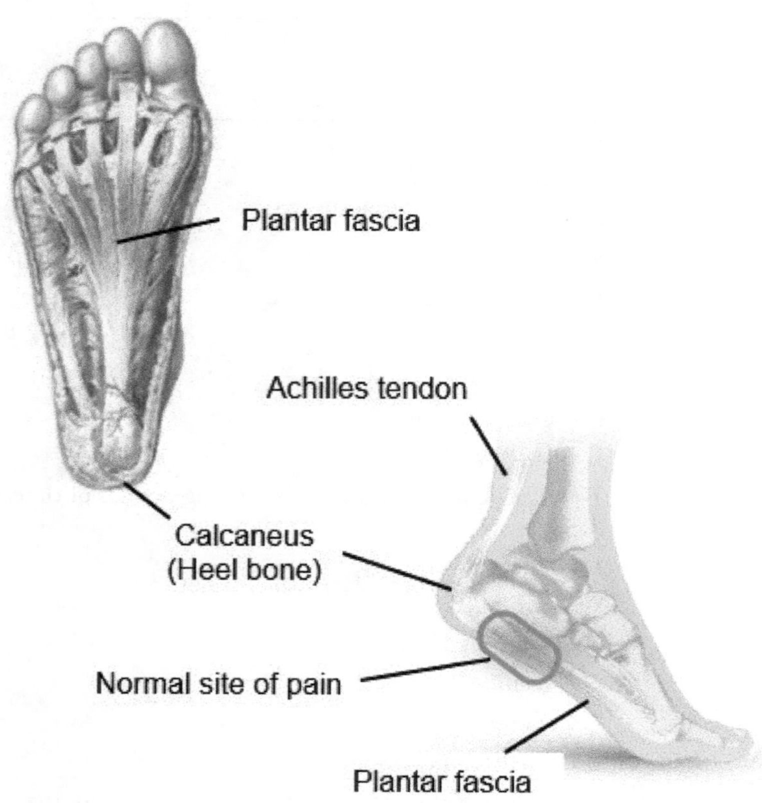

Figure 21.3 Plantar fascia and plantar fasciitis.

Although PF usually resolves on its own in 6 -1 8 months, NSAIDS, orthotics, braces, and splints, and stretching and strengthening exercises may be recommended by a clinician. Because a tight gastrocnemius has been directly associated with PF, calf and hamstring stretching should begin early in intervention. Additionally, rolling the plantar fascia with a can at night and first thing in the morning for 1-3 minutes will help break fascia adhesions. If non-invasive therapies do not provide relief, surgical intervention may be necessary. Stability and mobility exercise should focus on balance and loosening the fascia, as well as strengthening the intrinsic foot muscles, while movement training should emphasize improving ADLs. Exercise guidelines are in Table 21.4.

Table 21.4

General activity guidelines for common injuries of the lower leg, ankle, and foot

Condition	Early intervention	Stability/mobility	Movement	Avoid
Shin splints	Rest Braces, supports, orthotics Taping Anti-inflammatories	Stretch the calf muscles for MTSS Stretch anterior tibialis for anterior shin splints Core strength and stability • Bridging • Bird dogs • Planks Knee strength and stability Balance progression	Movements should initially focus on ADLs Low-loaded Open kinetic chain Closed kinetic chain Low impact cardio Pool-based activity Stationary bicycle	Repetitive loading High-impact landing Inversion

Ankle sprains	RICE Tapping, bracing, wrapping Progressive weight bearing for Grades I & II	Only perform if there is NO PAIN. Foot and ankle ROM (dorsiflexion, plantar flexion, inversion, eversion) Calf stretching OKC ankle movements with a band (dorsiflexion, plantar flexion, inversion, eversion) CKC movements Straight leg and bent leg calf raises Towel crunches with toes Marble pick up with toes Wobble board balance Balance progression	Single leg movements Reintroduce multiplanar-movements Leg press Wall squats Side steps Low impact cardiovascular training, progressed to higher intensity activity	Multiplanar-movements High impact
Achilles tendinopathy	Rest Oral or injectable anti-inflammatories, Weight-loss, Assessment of footwear Orthotics Assessment of body mechanics Physical therapy	Posterior chain stretching below pain tolerance Bi-lateral and unilateral heel drops Balance progression	Closed kinetic chain eccentric exercises • Leg press • Wall squats • Side steps Eccentric, and fast-rebounding heel-rises with increasing speed, ROM, and reps	Jumping Running Stairs
Plantar fasciitis	Rest NSAIDS Night splints Bracing orthotics	Balance progression Calf and hamstring flexibility SMR plantar fascia Towel scrunching Marble pick up	ADLs Toe curls Ankle circles	Running Jumping Stairs

Bolivar, et al., 2013; Cheatham, 2015; Galbraith & Lavallee, 2009; Kaminski et al., 2013; Memorial Sloan Kettering Cancer Center, 2019; Schwartz & Su, 2014; Silbernagel, Brorsson, & Lundberg, 2011; Sussmilch-Leitch et al., 2012; van den Bekerom et al., 2013

Discussion and application

1. What are some common lower leg injuries associated with pes planus, pes cavus, tight calf muscles, and/or excessive pronation? Describe the mechanisms of the injury and the treatment protocols.

References

American Academy of Orthopaedic Surgeons. (2019). Diseases and conditions: Sprained ankle. Orthoinfo. Retrieved from https://orthoinfo.aaos.org/en/diseases--conditions/sprained-ankle/

Bolivar, Y. A., Munuera, P. V., & Padillo, J. P. (2013). Relationship between tightness of the posterior muscles of the lower limb and plantar fasciitis. *Foot Ankle International, 34*(1), 42-48. https://doi.org/10.1177/1071100712459173

Cheatham, S. (2015). Musculoskeletal injuries of the lower extremity in J.S. Skinner, C.X. Bryant, S. Merrill, & D.J. Green (Eds), *American Council on Exercise medical exercise specialist manual.* San Diego, CA: American Council on Exercise.

Galbraith, R. M., & Lavallee, M. E. (2009). Medial tibial stress syndrome: Conservative treatment options. *Current Reviews in Musculoskeletal Medicine, 2*(3), 127-133. https://doi.org/10.1007/s12178-009-9055-6

Kaminski, T. W., Hertel, J., Amendola, N., Docherty, C. L., Dolan, M. G., Hopkins, J. T.,...Richie, D. (2013). National Athletic Trainers' Association position statement: Conservative management and prevention of ankle sprains in athletes. *Journal of Athletic Training, 48*(4), 528-545. https://doi.org/10.4085/1062-6050-48.4.02

Kirby, K. A. (2017). Longitudinal arch load-sharing system of the foot. *Revista Española de Podología, 28*(1), e18-e26. doi:1ttps://doi.org/0.1016/j.repod.2017.03.003

Lemme, N. J., Li, N. Y., DeFroda, S. F., Kleiner, J., & Owens, B. D. (2018). Epidemiology of Achilles tendon ruptures in the United States: Athletic and nonathletic injuries from 2012 to 2016. *Orthopaedic Journal of Sports Medicine, 6(*11), 2325967118808238. https://doi.org/10.1177/2325967118808238

Mandom, S., & Paul, J. (2015). Effectiveness of stretching and modified footwear on reducing pain and functional ability in athletes suffering from shin splint. International *Journal of Medical and Exercise Science, 1*(1), 16-21. Retrieved from http://www.ijmaes.org

Ott, S. M. (2013). Common ankle injuries [PowerPoint slides]. Retrieved from http://forms.acsm.org/tpc/PDFs/7%20Ott.pdf

Schwartz, E. N., & Su, J. (2014). Plantar fasciitis: A concise review. *The Permanente Journal, 18*(1), e105-107. https://doi.org/10.7812/TPP/13-113

Shah, S., Thomas, A. C., Noone, J. M., Blanchette, C. M., & Wikstrom, E. A. (2016). Incidence and cost of ankle sprains in United States emergency departments. *Sports Health, 8*(6), 547-552. https://doi.org/10.1177/1941738116659639

Shamrock, A. G. & Varacallo M. (2019). *Achilles tendon ruptures.* In: *StatPearls* [Internet]. Treasure Island, FL: StatPearls Publishing. Retrieved from https://www.ncbi.nlm.nih.gov/books/NBK430844/

Silbernagel, K. G., Brorsson, A., & Lundberg, M. (2011). The majority of patients with Achilles tendinopathy recover fully when treated with exercise alone: A 5-year follow-up. *American Journal of Sports Medicine, 39*(3), 607-613. https://doi.org/10.1177/0363546510384789

Sussmilch-Leitch, S. P., Collins, N. J., Bialocerkowski, A. E., Warden, S. J., & Crossley, K. M. (2012). Physical therapies for Achilles tendinopathy: Systematic review and meta-analysis. *Journal of Foot and Ankle Research, 5*(1), 1-16. https://doi.org/10.1186/1757-1146-5-15.

van den Bekerom, M. P., Kerkhoffs, G. M., McCollum, G. A., Calder, J. D., & van Dijk, C. N. (2013). Management of acute lateral ankle ligament injury in the athlete. *Knee Surgery, Sports Traumatology, Arthroscopy, 21*(6), 1390-1395. https://doi.org/10.1007/s00167-012-2252-7

CHAPTER 22
LOW BACK PAIN

By the end of this chapter you will understand:

- Prevalence and definition
- Pathophysiology of low back pain
- Factors leading to low back pain
- Treatment protocols
    - o Education
    - o Pharmacology and surgical intervention
    - o Exercise
- Core musculature and stabilization
- Exercise progression and examples

The Prevalence of Low Back Pain

Back pain is the leading cause of disability worldwide, and an estimated 80% of adults will suffer from low back pain (LBP) during their lifetime. In the United States, back pain accounts for more than 264 million lost workdays per year, and is thought to cost over $100 billion per year in lost wages, lost productivity, and increased healthcare costs (American Chiropractic Association, 2019; National Institute of Neurological Disorders and Stroke, 2019). Risk factors for LBP are age, sex, height, weight, sedentary lifestyle, depression, anxiety, insomnia, and smoking (Sharp, 2018). Fortunately, most patients require minimal treatment for recovery, and most LBP can be relieved once an underlying cause is treated (American College of Sports Medicine [ACSM], 2018; Casazza, 2012). However, to stay within a fitness professionals' scope of practice it is important to understand the various causes of LBP. LBP is defined as localized pain or ache below the costal margin (lower edge of the chest) and above the gluteal folds (below the buttocks but above the thigh) as shown in Figure 22.1. Acute LBP is pain generally experienced for 6–12 weeks, and chronic LBP is pain experienced for greater than 12 weeks (Sharp, 2018; Wheeler et al., 2017).

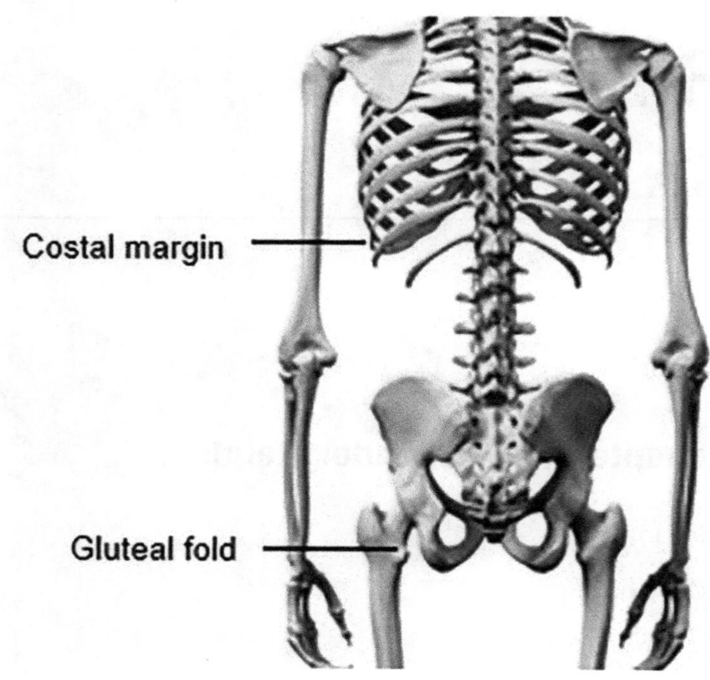

Figure 22.1 Low back pain is pain that occurs anywhere from the costal margin to the gluteal fold.

Although muscle strain and imbalance, ligament sprain, and soft tissue damage account for almost all LBP, often times the pain is non-specific, meaning it has no identifiable underlying condition or origin (Solomon, 2015; Wheeler et al., 2017). Because the core is a complex structure of spinal components, discs, intervertebral joints, muscles, and nerves, LBP can present with the same symptoms for different causes it is important to recognize the etiology. However, if a client presents with any type of back pain, it is strongly suggested the client be referred to a physician for a thorough exam prior to an exercise intervention. Table 22.1 details some differential diagnoses and key displays of LBP.

Table 22.1

Conditions, signs, and symptoms associated with low back pain

Condition	Cause	Signs/Symptoms
Abdominal aortic aneurysm*	Weak spot in the aorta/smoking	Abdominal discomfort/pulsating abdominal mass
Arthritis	Various	Morning stiffness/improves with activity
Compression fracture	History of trauma	Spinal tenderness/pain with flexion/and some movements

Discogenic back pain	Degeneration caused by age, obesity, smoking, excessive axial loading, resulting in reduced water in the disc nucleus	Inflammation /pain increases with forward flexion, sitting, or coughing/ Spinal instability/ limited controlled spinal mobility
Herniated disc	A portion of the nucleus pushes through a crack in the annulus	Pain mostly in leg, but also in back, radiating below the knee
Lumbar sprain/strain	Poor mechanics/over activity	Diffuse back and buttock pain that worsens with movement and is alleviated with rest
Metastatic cancer	Cancer	Sudden severe pain/spinal instability
Pelvic/renal/gastrointestinal issues	Various	Abdominal distress or pain/nausea/vomiting/ abnormal urinalysis
Sciatica	90% caused by a herniated disc Up to 6% caused by nerve impingement by the piriformis	Radicular pain down the thigh to the lower leg and foot
Spinal cord compression	Herniated disc	Pain/weakness/motor control dysfunction
Spinal stenosis	Thickening of the ligament in flavum (bands that cover the spinal canal)	Pain in the calf and distal lower extremity that may be alleviated when flexed or seated/sensory loss/weakness in the legs
Spondylosis	Degeneration of disc or facet arthropathy caused by repetitive impact or hyperextension	Disc pain worsens with flexion and sitting/facet pain worsens with extension/standing/walking
Spondylolisthesis (fractured vertebra)	Slipping of the vertebra relative to the one below it, caused by repetitive impact or hyperextension	Pain mostly in leg, but also in back, which worsens with standing and walking/is alleviated with rest
Vertebral osteomyelitis or infection	Spinal trauma/bacteria in intervertebral disc space	Gradual onset of pain, becoming constant /fever

Casazza, 2012; Hu, Tribus, Diab, & Ghanayem, 2008; Hicks, & Varacallo, 2018; Kinkade, 2007; Solomon, 2015; Wheeler et al., 2017

*This is considered a medical emergency

Treatment Protocols

Education

Even though the primary treatment goal for LBP is to relieve pain and improve activities of daily living (ADLs), the chance of recurrence is as high as 60% in the first year. Education along with an active recovery plan is the generally accepted protocol (ACSM, 2018; Solomon, 2015). Education should focus on psychosocial aspects of manageing chronic pain such as encouraging activities, and discouraging bed rest, as well as reassuring the client the condition can improve. Education also needs to address misconceptions regarding LBP as there is little evidence to support back exercises and general stretching alleviates LBP, and because each client situation is different, there is no standard protocol or template for assessment or treatment (McGill, n.d; Sharp, 2018).

Pharmacology and surgery

Pharmacological therapies include NSIADs for acute LBP, as well as some narcotics and muscle relaxers. Medications that act on the central nervous system can be used for neuropathy or to assist in nerve stabilization. Steroid and local anesthesia injections may relive pain and inflammation and allow less invasive therapies such as physical therapy to progress (Solomon, 2015). If conservative treatments do not relieve the symptoms, surgery may be necessary. Procedures such as a laminectomy or discectomy can be performed to relieve compression or impingement, and spinal fusion can be performed to stabilize degenerated discs.

Exercise

Because 97% of LPB is due to muscle strain, ligament sprain, and soft tissue damage, exercise is the primary means of treatment. Additionally, because core muscle activity is known to be dysfunctional in patients with LBP, early intervention should focus on re-education of faulty motor patterns through core activation, keeping in mind the muscles of the core function differently than muscles that control extremities (ACSM, 2018; Dalcourt & Comana, 2015; McGill, 2010). Because the spine is inherently unstable, core muscles co-contract and act in concert as synergists, and therefore need to be trained differently than muscles that control extremities (Faries & Greenwood, 2007; McGill, 2010). Local muscles are generally shorter than global muscles, attach to the spine, and are used mostly to provide segmental stability; whereas, global muscles (remember the slings from Chapter 16) produce speed and power, function in multiple planes of motions, and transfer loads to and from the extremities (Faries & Greenwood, 2007). Table 22.2 details core muscles and their actions.

Table 22.2

Core musculature and movements

Local muscles—Stabilization	Action	Global muscles—Mobilization	Action
Transversus abdominis	Draws abdominal wall to the spine, helps maintain abdominal pressure	Rectus abdominis	Flexes vertebral column
Multifidi	Extension, contraction, and rotation of vertebral column	Lateral fibers of external oblique	Helps increase intra-abdominal pressure
Internal oblique	Helps with respiration, aids in raising abdominal pressure, helps with truck rotation	Psoas major	Assists with the flexion and external rotation of the hip

Medial fibers of external oblique	Helps with ipsilateral side-bending and contralateral rotation	Erector spinae	Extension of vertebral column
Quadratus lumborum	Helps with extension and lateral flexion of the vertebral column	Iliocostalis (thoracic portion)	Extends and laterally flexes the thoracic spine
Diaphragm	Through contraction and relaxation, alters the volume of the thoracic cavity and lungs, producing inspiration and expiration	Longissimus thoracis	Flexion and extension of vertebral column
Iliocostalis and longissimus (lumbar portions)	Helps with posture, transfers loads, stabilizes the spine for flexion and extension		
Thoracolumbar fascia	Supports vertebral column flexion via fascial tension		
Intertransversarii	Proprioception		
Interspinales	Proprioception		
Rotatores	Proprioception		

ACSM, 2018; Donatelli, 2007; Faries & Greenwood, 2007

The goal of exercise treatment for LBP is to alleviate pain, restore spinal stability, and help a client return to normal ADLs. The first step is to remove the cause of pain, or faulty movement patterns. Although each client situation is different, there are a number of concepts that apply universally (McGill, 2010; Solomon, 2015):

- Many back injuries are the result of cumulative trauma rather than a single event.
- Individuals with a greater range of motion of the back are at a greater risk for LBP.
- Most back injuries result in spinal instability; therefore, exercises to enhance spinal stability and posture may be the best intervention for acute LBP.
- A greater degree of back strength does not equate to back health and has not been shown to be of more benefit for clients who suffer from LBP; endurance of the back muscles is more important.
- Due to excessive forward flexion and a high degree of spinal loading, sit-ups may induce LBP.
- A combination of low intensity activity, such as walking, coupled with condition-specific back exercises offers the best results for resolution and prevention of LBP.

- Due to osmotic hydration, vertebral discs are more hydrated in the morning following bed rest, and more susceptible to injury, particularly during forward flexion.
- The first time a new movement is performed it should be considered an assessment. If it causes pain, adjust the movement as needed.
- Although most exercise plans are programed for 2–3 days per week, core training can be performed daily.

Exercise treatment for LBP should start with correcting faulty motor patterns, followed by increasing muscular endurance, then strength and power. To accomplish this, the following training progression is suggested, and examples of exercises for each stage are in Table 22.3.

1. Corrective, therapeutic, and perfect motion motor patterns exercise as determined by the initial assessment.
    a. Identify and remove movements that cause pain.
    b. Ensure proper posture and gluteal activation during ADLs.
    c. Form, form, form.
    d. Perform abdominal bracing to encourage co-contraction (not to be confused with abdominal hollowing that may be counterproductive as it engages only one or two core muscles).
2. Build whole-body and joint stability (mobility at some joints such as the hips and stability through the lumbar/core region).
    a. These exercises increase stability without exacerbating the original injury.
    b. These movements should challenge endurance and increase motor control.
    c. Bracing and co-contraction of the core should be performed during these movements.
3. Increase endurance.
    a. Isometrics should be held for less than10 seconds; to increase endurance, increase repetitions.
    b. A pyramid pattern (5 reps on each side, 4 reps, 3 reps, 2 reps, 1 rep) allows the most repetitions to be performed with the least fatigue.

For occupational/athletic clients:

4. Build strength.
    a. Build on an achieved foundation.
    b. Match skills and exercises with abilities and ADLs.
5. Develop speed, power, and agility.
    a. Power requires a stiff torso with relaxed (not to be confused with loose) extremities.
    b. Focus should be on required performance movements.

Table 22.3

Example exercises for low back pain

Corrective and Therapeutic	Whole body—joint stability	Endurance	Strength	Power	Avoid (until appropriately progressed)
Abdominal bracing Wall roll Floor roll Glute bridges Clamshell Single leg squat matrix Low-load cardio-vascular exercise such as walking	Cat-camel stretch Modified curl up Opposite arm/leg raise Quadruped bird-dog Side bridge/modified Plank Rolling bridge Push-ups Modified Staggered hands Unstable surface Body rows	Start with 0-10 second isometrics Increase the number of reps not the length of the isometric hold A pyramid pattern can provide ample repetitions as well as ample rest	Focus on ADLs Unilateral farmers walk Lateral cable hold-press	Plyometrics Medicine ball slams Whirling m/b to slams Medicineball catch	Heavy lifting Prolonged sitting Twisting movements

McGill, 2010, Solomon, 2015

Discussion and application

1. Discuss different types/causes of LBP, and what are risk factors associated with LBP?
2. What are some common misconceptions regarding exercise treatment for LBP?
3. Design a program for an individual experiencing LBP. Discuss the progressions and provide example exercises.

References

American Chiropractic Association. (2019). Back pain facts and statistics. Retrieved from https://www.acatoday.org/Patients/Health-Wellness-Information/Back-Pain-Facts-and-statistics

American College of Sports Medicine. (2018). *ACSM's resources for the exercise physiologist: A practical guide for the health fitness professional* (P. Magyari, R. Lite, M. W. Kilpatrick, & J. E. Schoffstall Eds. 2 ed.). Philadelphia, PA: Wolters Kluwer.

Casazza, B. A. (2012). Diagnosis and treatment of acute low back pain. *American Family Physician, 85*(4), 343-350. Retrieved from http://www.aafp.org/afp/2012/0215/p343.html

Dalcourt, M., & Comana, F. (2015). Balance and gait in J.S. Skinner, C.X. Bryant, S. Merrill, & D.J. Green (Eds), *American Council on Exercise medical exercise specialist manual.* San Diego, CA: American Council on Exercise.

Donatelli, R. A. (2007). The anatomy and pathophysiology of the core. In R. A. Donatelli (Ed.), *Sports-specific rehabilitation* (pp. 135-143). St. Louis, MO: Churchill Livingstone, Elsevier Inc.

Faries, M. D., & Greenwood, M. (2007). Core training: Stabilizing the confusion. *Strength and Conditioning Journal, 29*(2), 10. https://doi.org/10.1519/00126548-200704000-00001

Hicks, B. L., & Varacallo, M. (2018). *Piriformis Syndrome* in StatPearls [Internet]. Treasure Island, FL: StatPearls Publishing. Retrieved from https://www.ncbi.nlm.nih.gov/books/NBK448172/

Hu, S. S., Tribus, C. B., Diab, M., & Ghanayem, A. J. (2008). Spondylolisthesis and spondylolysis. *The Journal of Bone & Joint Surgery, 90A*(3), 656-671. Retrieved from http://journals.lww.com/jbjsjournal/toc/2008/03000

Kinkade, S. (2007). Evaluation and treatment of acute low back pain. *American Family Physician, 75*, 1181-1188. Retrieved from http://www.aafp.org/afp/2007/0415/p1181.html

McGill, S. (n.d.). Designing back exercise: From rehabilitation to enhancing performance. *Backfitpro.* Retrieved from http://www.backfitpro.com/articles.php

McGill, S. M. (2010). Core training: Evidence translating to better performance and injury prevention. *Strength & Conditioning Journal, 32*(3), 33-46. https://doi.org/10.1519/SSC.0b013e3181df4521

National Institute of Neurological Disorders and Stroke. (2019). Low back pain fact sheet. Retrieved from https://www.ninds.nih.gov/disorders/patient-caregiver-education/fact-sheets/low-back-pain-fact-sheet

Sharp, C. (2018). Musculoskeletal conditions and disorders in P.L. Jacobs (Ed) *NSCA's essentials of training special populations.* Champaign, IL: Human Kinetics

Soloman, J. (2015). Low back pain in J.S. Skinner, C.X. Bryant, S. Merrill, & D.J. Green (Eds), *American Council on Exercise medical exercise specialist manual.* San Diego, CA: American Council on Exercise.

Wheeler, S. G., Wipf, J. E., Staiger, T. O., Deyo, R. A., & Jarvik, J. G. (2017). Evaluation of low back pain in adults. In S.J. Atlas (ed.) *UpToDate.* Retrieved April 13, 2020 from https://www.uptodate.com/contents/evaluation-of-low-back-pain-in-adults

CHAPTER 23
ARTHRITIS

By the end of this chapter you will understand:

- Type and epidemiology
  - o Osteoarthritis
  - o Rheumatoid arthritis
- Diagnostic criteria/presentation
- Treatment options
  - o Nutrition
  - o Pharmacological
  - o Exercise
- Exercise guidelines

Background

Arthritis is a family of more than 100 diseases including osteoarthritis (OA), rheumatoid arthritis (RA), gout, fibromyalgia, lupus, and scleroderma. Arthritis is the leading disability in the United States, affecting almost 55 million adults, and costing over $30 billion annually in health care costs, lost wages, and lost productivity. By conservative estimates, close to 60% of individuals over the age of 60 have some form of arthritis, as do 1/3 of individuals age 18-64 (Arthritis Foundation, n.d.). Primary risk factors include female sex, age, race, and structural malalignment. Secondary risk factors include prior trauma, physically demanding job, muscle weakness, and metabolic disease (Sharp, 2018). Comorbidities include obesity, diabetes, anxiety and depression, and heart disease. The good news is exercise and physical activity can improve physical function by about 40%.

Osteoarthritis

OA is the most prevalent joint disease in the United States affecting close to 30 million adults (Arthritis Foundation, n.d.). OA is degenerative and characterized by pain, swelling, joint stiffness, and decreased strength, flexibility, and cardiorespiratory capacity (American College of Sports Medicine [ACSM], 2018). OA occurs when the cartilage and synovial fluid that cushions and lubricates bones and joints are lost. As cartilage breaks down, the connecting bone also wears down due to constant rubbing, which can lead to bone spurs. As cartilage and bone wear away, small pieces can chip off and get caught in the joint, creating more wear and tear, inflammation, swelling, and pain (Arthritis Foundation, n.d.). OA mostly effects large, weight bearing joints (knees, hips, and spine) but can also occur in the fingers and toes. The American College of Rheumatology suggests the presence of persistent knee pain, limited morning stiffness, and reduced function, coupled with crepitus, restricted movement, and bony enlargement predicts with 99% accuracy a correct diagnosis of OA (Heidari, 2011). Table 23.1 provides more detail for the American College of Rheumatology criteria for a diagnosis of knee OA.

Table 23.1

American College of Rheumatology criteria for the diagnosis of knee OA

Clinical process	Criteria	Symptoms
Using history and clinical examination	Pain in the knee and three of the following symptoms:	Age >50 years
		Morning stiffness <30 minutes
		Crepitus on active motions
		Bony tenderness
		Bony enlargement
		No palpable warmth of synovium
Using history and clinical examination and radiographic findings	Pain in the knee and one of the following symptoms:	Age >50 years
		Morning stiffness < 30 minutes
		Crepitus on active motions and osteophyte
Using history and clinical examination and laboratory findings	Pain in the knee and 5 of the following symptoms:	Age >50 years
		Morning stiffness <30 minutes
		Crepitus on active motions
		Bony enlargement
		No palpable warmth of synovium
		ESR <40 mm/h
		Rheumatoid Factor <1/40
		Synovial fluid signs of osteoarthritis

Aronen & Lorenz, 2015; Heidari, 2011

Pharmacology

OA has no cure, so management of pain, inflammation, and joint stiffness, as well as slowing progression are the goals of pharmacological treatment. Over the counter (OTC) non-steroidal anti-inflammatories (NSAIDS) and acetaminophen products can reduce pain and swelling; however side effects can include gastrointestinal problems or cardiovascular events (Aronen & Lorenz, 2015; Sharp, 2018). Topical pain relievers such as menthol and capsaicin can provide nominal pain relief with minimal side effects. Prescription NSAIDs reduce inflammation and pain to a greater degree than OTC products, but increase the risk of heart attack or stroke. Corticosteroids are usually prescribed when NSAIDs and other oral pain relievers are ineffective. Corticosteroids are injected directly into the joint to reduce inflammation, but over the long term, in large doses, can cause osteoporosis via inhibition of osteoblast activity. Viscosupplements are injected directly into the joint to replace lost fluids and increase lubrication and can be injected as needed. Narcotics are only used when the pain becomes unbearable, but caution should be used to avoid dependency, and increasing tolerance (Sharp, 2018). Drugs used for OA treatment, their actions, and side effects are presented in Table 23.2.

Table 23.2

Pharmacology used for the treatment of OA

Drug/Type	Action	Side effects
OTC NSAIDS and acetaminophen	Reduce pain and swelling	gastrointestinal problems or cardiovascular events
Topical pain relievers such as menthol and capsaicin	Pain relief	Minimal
Prescription NSAIDs	Reduce inflammation and pain	increase the risk of heart attack or stroke
Corticosteroids	Reduce inflammation	but over the long term, in large doses, can cause osteoporosis
Viscosupplements	Replace lost fluids and increase lubrication	Temporary
Narcotics	Pain relief	Addiction

Aronen & Lorenz, 2015; Sharp, 2018

Nutritional supplements

Many nutritional supplements can also be purchased OTC. Glucosamine and chondroitin can alleviate inflammation and may stimulate cartilage production. Omega-3 fatty acids are known to reduce joint swelling, pain, and the duration of morning joint stiffness by inhibiting the expression and production of inflammatory processes, and increasing anti-inflammatory mechanisms (Calder, 2012). While Omega-3 fatty acids provide an anti-inflammatory response, Omega-6 fatty acids are considered pro-inflammatory and should be avoided or moderated (Aronen & Lorenz, 2015; Calder, 2012). Other nutrients that may minimize the inflammatory effects of OA are antioxidants, methylsulfonylmethane (MSM) may decrease swelling and pain by replacing lost sulfur in the joints, hyaluronan may help prevent soft-tissue damage by restoring water into the extracellular matrix, and pro- and pre-biotics can increase the immune response by supplying the gut with healthy bacteria and yeast (Aronen & Lorenz, 2015). Please keep in mind it is beyond the scope of practice for a CXS to prescribe supplements or pharmacological agents to any client. Nutritional supplements used for the treatment of OA and their actions are found in Table 23.3.

Table 23.3

Nutritional supplements used for the treatment of OA

Supplement	Action
Glucosamine and chondroitin	Alleviates inflammation Stimulates cartilage production
Omega-3 fatty acids	Anti-inflammatory properties reduce joint swelling
Antioxidants	Anti-inflammatory properties reduce joint swelling
Methylsulfonylmethane (MSM	Decreases swelling and pain by replacing lost sulfur
Hyaluronan	Restores water into the extracellular matrix
Pro- and pre-biotics	Increases the immune response
Aronen & Lorenz, 2015; Calder, 2012	

Exercise intervention

Quality of life is the objective of exercise therapy for clients with OA as exercise can reduce joint pain, improve physical functioning, and alleviate systemic inflammation often found with comorbidities such as obesity, cardiovascular disease (CVD), and Type II diabetes (Dressendorfer, 2017). Unfortunately, there is no consensus on exercise recommendations for OA; however, some elements are consistent in the literature. Exercise for cardiovascular conditioning, strength development, flexibility, and neuromuscular control such as Tai Chi or yoga should be incorporated into an OA exercise program (ACSM, 2018; Aronen & Lorenz, 2015; Dressendorfer, 2017; Sharp, 2018). The low to moderate intensity of Tai Chi and yoga, coupled with the cardiovascular and strength benefits, as well as improvements in balance, pain, fatigue, stiffness, and reduced stress, suggest neuromuscular training may be particularly beneficial for deconditioned clients (Field, 2016; Lan, Chen, & Lai, 2008; Larson-Meyer, 2016). Table 23.5 combines the recommendations of a number of organizations. Additionally, the following contraindications and precautions should be considered before an exercise program (Aronen & Lorenz, 2015; Dressendorfer, 2017):

- All comorbidities should be evaluated separately and considered for any exercise contraindications and recommendations.
- Activities that increase or exacerbate pain should be avoided.
- During acute flare-ups, intense exercise should be avoided, but mild activity such as range of motion exercises are encouraged.
- Assure clients that some pain while exercising is normal.
- Balance and gait can be affected by OA in the lower extremities placing clients at an increased risk for falling.
- An adequate warm-up should be performed to increase joint lubrication and tissue elasticity.
- Aerobic exercise to increase endurance and cardiovascular capacity should be suggested prior to a combined program of aerobic and resistance exercise.
- Exercising in a warm pool, 86-88 degrees °F, will relax muscles and reduce pain.

- Higher intensity is not necessarily more effective than low intensity to reduce pain and improve physical function.
- Obese clients should be encouraged to perform low-intensity exercise with more repitions.
- The protocols and exercises for clients with similar orthopedic dysfunctions (Chapters 17-22) should be considered.

Rheumatoid Arthritis

RA is the most common autoimmune disorder causing chronic joint inflammation, pain, stiffness, and warmth in an affected area (Melrose, Dawes, Kesterson, & Reuter, 2018). The immune system mistakenly attacks joint tissue, synovial lining, and cartilage, causing the joint lining to thicken. RA is most common in the wrists, fingers, and hands, but may progress to the elbows, knees, and ankles (Arthritis Foundation, n.d.). Diagnostic criteria for RA include the number of affected joints, the extent of swelling, the presence of RA antibodies, and duration of symptoms. RA is considered a systemic disease as it may also affect other systems of the body including the cardiovascular, respiratory, and renal (Melrose, et al., 2018).

It is estimated RA affects up to 1.5 million people, with an associated annual cost of $39.2 billion. RA affects women at twice the rate of men, and mortality hazards are 60-70% higher in patients with RA compared with people in the general population (Arthritis Foundation, n.d.). Risk factors include a genetic history, age, smoking, stress, obesity, previous infections, and diet. Comorbidities are similar to those associated with OA, but also include asthma, malignancies, and chronic obstructive pulmonary disorder (Dougados et al., 2014). Additionally, it is suggested the incidence of CVD for an individual with RA is similar to individuals with Type II diabetes, and CVD may account for the increased mortality rate and be considered an independent risk factor for inflammatory arthritis. Equally, smoking is the single most preventable risk factor and accounts for up to as much as 25% the burden of RA. Suggestions for the management of CVD in patients with RA include:

- RA should be regarded as a condition associated with higher risk for CVD. The increased risk appears to be due to both an increased prevalence of traditional risk factors and the inflammatory burden
- Adequate control of disease activity is necessary to lower the CVD risk
- A CVD risk assessment is recommended for all patients with RA
- RA patients should consider quitting smoking (Peters et al., 2010)

Pharmacology

Pharmacological therapy for RA is similar to that for OA with the addition of disease-modifying antirheumatic drugs (DMARDs). DMARDs can be taken alone, or with NSAIDs, corticosteroids, or biologic response modifiers. DMARDs are immunosuppressants and place a client at an increased risk for infections, whereas biologic response modifiers increase the body's response to infection (Melrose et al., 2018). It is important to speak with a client's physician to be aware of any adverse side effects or contraindications to exercise because of pharmacological therapy.

Nutrition

The reduction of unhealthy gut microbiota is a main goal of dietary intervention for RA. Various diets, as well as individual foods and supplements can reduce inflammation, conversely, other foods may aggravate the condition and should be avoided. The following are some examples of beneficial diets (Khanna, Jaiswal, & Gupta, 2017):

- Fasting for 7 days followed by a vegan diet for a year may reduce joint swelling and tenderness.
- A vegan diet that eliminates any animal product or by product, has been shown to eliminate antigens that instigate immune reactive responses.
- A Mediterranean diet, high in Omega-3 fatty acids, fruits, vegetables, legumes, and low in red meat, has been shown to reduce inflammation, and improve quality of life.
- An elimination diet focuses on reducing foods that aggravate symptoms.

Because the details of specific diets are beyond the scope of this text, a client's physician and/or registered dietician should be consulted prior to making dietary changes. See Table 23.4 for a list of foods that may help with or exacerbate RA symptoms.

Table 23.4

Foods that may help with, exacerbate RA symptoms

Food	Characteristic	Benefit	Detriment
Whole grains	Dietary fiber antioxidants, phytic acid, vitamin E, selenium	Aids in digestion and the formation of beneficial microflora Anti-inflammatory	
Fruits	Bioactive components and phytochemicals	Antioxidant Anti-inflammatory	
Ginger	Phenolic acids	Reduces nausea, pain, and inflammation.	
Turmeric/Curcumin	Phenolic acids	Antioxidant Anti-inflammatory	
Cinnamon bark	Polyphenolic fraction	Aids in reducing GI distress Aids in recuing infections caused by bacteria and parasitic worms Appetite stimulant	
Omega-3		Immunosuppressant and anti-inflammatory	
Probiotics/Prebiotics	Bifdobacterium and Lactobacillus	Antioxidant	

Alcohol	No evidence to support the benefits or detriments		
Tea (Green)	Phytochemicals	Antioxidant Anti-inflammatory	
Hydrogenated Oils	Omega-6 fatty acid (non-GFLA)		Pro-inflammatory
Saturated fats	No double bonded molecules, saturated with hydrogen		Raises cholesterol Triggers adipose or fat tissue inflammation
Trans Fats	Hydrogenated oil		Triggers systemic inflammation
Red and Processed Meats	Contains hormones and fats		Triggers systemic inflammation
Refined sugars	Cytokines		Can cause inflammation by triggering an immune response
Gluten	Allergen		Can cause inflammation by triggering an immune response

Duckworth, 2018; Khanna, Jaiswal, & Gupta, 2017

Exercise intervention

In addition to reducing the effects of a sedentary lifestyle, exercise can reduce pain, joint stiffness, and fatigue in RA patients (ACSM, 2018). Reducing muscle atrophy via resistance training can hinder osteoporosis, and reduce the risk of falls, while aerobic training can reduce the risk of CVD, diabetes, and obesity, and stretching can alleviate joint pain and stiffness. Although performing activity can be painful, exercise can help with activities of daily living, improve sleep, fight fatigue, boost immunity, and improve emotional well-being. A combination of aerobic and resistance training has been proven to be the most beneficial. In addition to the benefits of neuromuscular training experienced by OA clients, including improvements in cardiovascular conditioning, strength, balance, reduced pain, fatigue, stiffness, and stress, RA clients can also realize reductions in cholesterol and inflammatory cytokines (Field, 2016; Lan, et al., 2008; Larson-Meyer, 2016). FITT recommendations for RA are similar to recommendations for OA, and are in Tables 23.5 and 23.6.

Table 23.5

FITT recommendations for OA

Condition	Frequency	Intensity	Time	Type
Aerobic	3-5 days/week	55-75% VO_2max 30-60% HRR RPE 9-13 The talk test may be best for deconditioned clients	Start with 5-15 min and progress to 30 minutes for a total of 150 min/week Multiple shorter sessions / day should be considered	Swimming Cycling Walking Rowing Arm ergometer
Resistance training	2-3 sessions/week of light to moderate intensity	40-60% 1RM Pain tolerance may have to be used as a guide	2-3 sets 6-8 reps 2-3 min of rest	Balance & Functional • Isometrics • Body weight • Bands • Dumbbells
Flexibility	3-7 days/week	Held to mild discomfort	3 sets 1-5 stretches/muscle group 5-30 sec. hold	Dynamic flexibility Static flexibility
Neuromuscular training	3-7 days/week	Up to 55% HRR	15 min progressing to 60 min	Pilates, yoga, tai chi,

ACSM, 2018; Aronen & Lorenz, 2015; Dressendorfer, 2017; Field, 2016; Lan, et al., 2008; Larson-Meyer, 2016; Melrose et al., 2018

Table 23.6

FITT recommendations for RA

Condition	Frequency	Intensity	Time	Type
Aerobic	Most days of the week	60-80%MHR 30-60% HRR	Start with short bouts, as tolerated, and progress to 150 min/week	Low impact Pool based exercise Biking Switch modes on consecutive days Can be combined with intermittent resistance training
Resistance	2-3 sessions/week of light to moderate intensity based on symptoms and tolerance	40-60% 1RM	8-12 full body movements Slowly progress to 3 sets of 10-15 reps	Body weight Bands Manual resistance (if qualified) Dumbbells
Flexibility	3-7 days/week	Held to mild discomfort	Static stretching hold for up to 30 sec. 3 reps each stretch	Dynamic flexibility Static flexibility

Neuromuscular training	3-7/days/week	Up to 55% HRR	15 min progressing to 60 min	Pilates, yoga, tai chi,

ACSM, 2018; Aronen & Lorenz, 2015; Dressendorfer, 2017; Field, 2016; Lan, et al., 2008; Larson-Meyer, 2016; Melrose et al., 2018

Discussion and application

1. Discuss the types of arthritis and the diagnostic criteria for each.
2. What are the recommended exercise guidelines for someone with arthritis, and what are some contraindications?

References

American College of Sports Medicine. (2018). *ACSM's resources for the exercise physiologist: A practical guide for the health fitness professional* (P. Magyari, R. Lite, M. W. Kilpatrick, & J. E. Schoffstall Eds. 2 ed.). Philadelphia, PA: Wolters Kluwer.

Aronen, J. G. & Lorenz, K. A. (2015). Arthritis in J.S. Skinner, C.X. Bryant, S. Merrill, & D.J. Green (Eds*), American Council on Exercise medical exercise specialist manual.* San Diego, CA: American Council on Exercise.

Arthritis Foundation. (n.d.). Arthritis by the numbers: Book of trusted facts and figures. Retrieved from https://www.arthritis.org/Documents/Sections/About-Arthritis/arthritis-facts-stats-figures.pdf

Calder, P. C. (2013). Omega-3 polyunsaturated fatty acids and inflammatory processes: Nutrition or pharmacology? *British Journal of Clinical Pharmacology, 75*(3), 645-662. https://doi.org/10.1111/j.1365-2125.2012.04374.x

Dougados, M., Soubrier, M., Antunez, A., Balint, P., Balsa, A., Buch, M. H.,...Kay, J. (2014). Prevalence of comorbidities in rheumatoid arthritis and evaluation of their monitoring: Results of an international, cross-sectional study (COMORA). *Annals of the Rheumatic Diseases, 73*(1), 62-68. https://doi.org/10.1136/annrheumdis-2013-204223

Dressendorfer, R. (2017). Exercise prescription for osteoarthritis. In S. Richman, (Ed.). *Cinahl Information System.* Glendale, CA: EBSCO Publishing.

Duckworth, H. (2018). RA inflammatory foods: What foods should I avoid? Retrieved from https://www.rheumatoidarthritis.org/living-with-ra/diet/inflammatory-foods/

Field, T. (2016). Tai Chi research review. *Journal of Complementary Medicine & Alternative Healthcare, 1*(1), 1-16. Retrieved from https://juniperpublishers.com/jcmah/

Heidari, B. (2011). Knee osteoarthritis diagnosis, treatment and associated factors of progression: Part II. *Caspian Journal of Internal Medicine, 2(*3), 249-255. Retrieved from https://europepmc.org/articles/PMC3770501;jsessionid=6592D35BEA4F2675B016AAF0D0A84BBC

Khanna, S., Jaiswal, K. S., & Gupta, B. (2017). Managing rheumatoid arthritis with dietary interventions. *Frontiers in Nutrition, 4*, 52. https://doi.org/10.3389/fnut.2017.00052

Lan, C., Chen, S., & Lai, J. (2008). The exercise intensity of Tai Chi Chuan. *Tai Chi Chuan: State of the Art in International Research, 52*, 12-19. https://doi.org/10.1159/000134225

Larson-Meyer, D. E. (2016). A systematic review of the energy cost and metabolic intensity of yoga. *Medicine & Science in Sports & Exercise, 48*(8), 1558-1569. https://doi.org/10.1249/mss.0000000000000922

Melrose, D., Dawes, J., Kesterson, M., & Reuter, B. (2018). Immunologic and hematologic disorders in P.L. Jacobs (Ed) *NSCA's essentials of training special populations*. Champaign, IL: Human Kinetics.

Peters, M. J., Symmons, D. P., McCarey, D., Dijkmans, B. A., Nicola, P., Kvien, T. K.,...Nurmohamed, M. T. (2010). EULAR evidence-based recommendations for cardiovascular risk management in patients with rheumatoid arthritis and other forms of inflammatory arthritis. *Annals of the Rheumatic Diseases, 69*(2), 325-331. https://doi.org/10.1136/ard.2009.113696

Sharp, C. (2018). Musculoskeletal conditions and disorders in P.L. Jacobs (Ed) *NSCA's essentials of training special populations*. Champaign, IL: Human Kinetics.

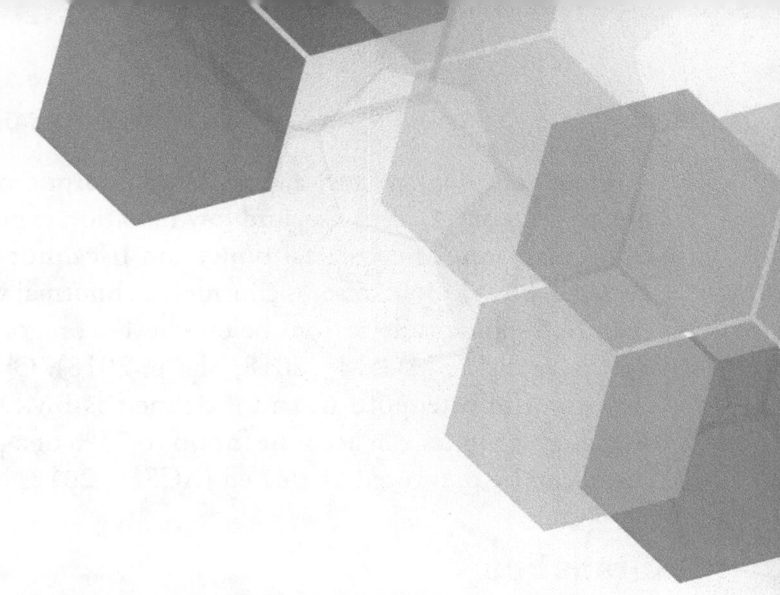

CHAPTER 24 OSTEOPOROSIS

By the end of this chapter you will understand:

- Statistics
- Mechanics of bone formation
- Factors that affect bone density
- The female triad
- Diagnostic criteria/presentation
- Treatment options
    - o Nutrition
    - o Pharmacological
    - o Exercise
- Preventive measures
- Exercise guidelines—FITT
- Contraindicated movements

Background

Osteoporosis is the most common bone disease in humans and is considered a major public health problem (Sozen, Ozisik, & Basaran, 2017). Osteoporosis is characterized by low bone mass, structural deterioration of the bone architecture in trabecular bone, and porous and thin cortical bone, resulting in decreased bone strength (Fletcher, 2013; Witzke, 2015). Although there are numerous methods to measure bone density, duel-energy X-ray absorptiometry (DEXA or DXA) is considered the gold-standard due to accuracy, ease of use, and low radiation exposure. However, DXA does not differentiate between trabecular bone and cortical bone, and it cannot determine bone architecture or material properties (Witzke, 2015). Bone mass is considered abnormal when bone mass density (BMD) is equal to, or greater than, 2.5 standard deviations below the T-score, or the young normal adult score (American College of Sports medicine [ACSM], 2018; Sharp, 2018). Osteopenia is also characterized by low BMD, but not the extent of osteoporosis, and is defined as BMD between 1.0 and 2.5 deviations below the T-score. Although genetics can account for up to 75% of a person's bone mineral density, osteoporosis, in many cases, can be prevented or treated (ACSM, 2018; National Institutes of Health, 2018).

Statistics

Osteoporosis affects over 10 million adults in the United States and almost 44 million have osteopenia. It is estimated by 2030 the combined number will increase to more than 71 million for adults over age 50 (National Osteoporosis Foundation, 2014). Females are at a higher risk than males, with 50% of females over age 50 afflicted, and 20% of males. Worldwide, there is a fracture associated with osteoporosis every 3 seconds, with the most frequent fractures in the hip, vertebrae, and wrist/forearm (International Osteoporosis Foundation, 2017; Witzke, 2015). Unfortunately, 25% of older adults who experience an osteoporotic fracture die within 5 years (ACSM, 2018). The associated annual cost of medical treatment and loss of productivity in the United States is estimated to be around $20 billion and is expected to increase to over $25 billion in the coming years (ACSM, 2018; Dempster, 2011).

Formation of Bone

Similar to other tissue, bone is in a constant state of remodeling, or breaking down and rebuilding. Osteoclasts breakdown bone matrix, while osteoblasts are responsible for repairing bone matrix. Osteoporosis results when the process of breaking down, or resorption, happens at a faster rate than reformation. Peak bone velocity and growth takes place in puberty, and peak bone mass occurs in early adulthood. It is shortly after peak bone mass, in the mid-twenties to early thirties that bone density starts to diminish in males, and early to mid-forties for females (ACSM, 2018; Sozen et al., 2017). Loss of bone mass stays at a steady rate for males but accelerates in females at the onset of menopause. Because peak bone velocity occurs during puberty, maximizing bone growth during this period will have positive health benefits in later years.

Factors That Effect Bone Mass Density

Factors that affect BMD are activity and exercise, nutrition, genetics, lifestyle, and disease (Gray, 2014; Mitchell, Cooper, Dawson-Hughes, Gordon, & Rizzoli, 2015; Sozen et al., 2017). Risk factors are classified into modifiable and non-modifiable. Non-modifiable factors cannot be changed and are usually genetic. Since the initial findings of the Human Genome Project in 2001, it is thought there are 20,500 human genes (National Human Genome Research Institute, 2018). Human genes are the coding of inheritable instructions for the next generation. Genome-wide association studies, and twin and family linkage studies have determined a genetic component associated with low BMD. Even though it is estimated up to 80% of risk for osteoporosis is genetic, the precise location of only a few genes has been found (Chesi et al, 2019; Marini, Masi, Marcucci, Cianferotti, & Brandi, 2018). Modifiable factors include, environment, diet, and activity level. Osteoporosis is classified as primary or secondary.

Primary osteoporosis, the most common, is age related and is the consequences of cumulative bone loss, and is non-modifiable. Secondary osteoporosis is the result of lifestyle or disease state, many of which are modifiable. Table 24.1 details risk factors, and some primary and secondary causes for osteoporosis.

Table 24.1

Osteoporosis risk factors, primary and secondary causes

Non-modifiable	Modifiable/Lifestyle	Disease Category
Female	Inactivity	Genetic • Cystic fibrosis • Marfan syndrome • Hemochromatosis
Age	Poor nutrition	Endocrine: • Central obesity • Diabetes • Athletic amenorrhea
Family history	Low calcium level	Gastrointestinal • Celiac disease • Gastric bypass/surgery • Pancreatic disease
Ethnicity (White, Asian)	Low Vitamin D level	Hematological • Leukemia • Hemophilia • Sickle Cell disease
Kyphosis	Excessive Vitamin A	Neurological • Epilepsy • Stroke • Parkinson's disease
Small body frame	Smoking	Musculoskeletal • Muscular dystrophy • Spinal cord injury • Proximal myopathy
Menopause prior to age 45	Excessive alcohol consumption	Autoimmune • Rheumatoid arthritis • HIV • Lupus
Previous fracture	Excessive soda	COPD
	Excessive caffeine	Depression
	Immobilization	Renal disease
	Low body weight	

	Fall risk • Impaired hearing • Impaired vision • Ill-fitting footwear and clothing • Poor ambulatory environment • Poor ambulatory environment
Chesi et al., 2019; Sharp, 2018; Sozen et al., 2017	

The Female Triad

A discussion of osteoporosis must include the female triad. The female triad is a syndrome characterized by low energy, amenorrhea, and osteoporosis (Barrack, Ackerman, & Gibbs, 2013). Even though all components may not be present, it is estimated 50-60% of female adolescent athletes have at least two components. Athletes involved in sports where a lean physique is preferred, such as figure skating and running, are the most vulnerable. Early detection and intervention are critical to avoid lifelong health concerns. The following risk factors should be assessed (Bush, 2018):

- Menstrual irregularities or amenorrhea
- History of stress facture
- A history of critical comments regarding food
- Depression
- Self-restricted food consumption
- Obsessiveness or perfectionism
- Weight fluctuations
- Overtraining
- Recurrent injuries
- Sleep disorders

Bone loss related to the female athlete triad is not fully understood. However, the most recent evidence suggests a combination of low estrogen levels and a chronic lack of proper nutrition leads to poor bone health and development (Witzke, 2015). Although further studies need to be conducted to clarify relationships, it is surmised low energy levels can result in weakening tissue such as muscles, tendons, and ligaments, leading to excessive musculoskeletal injuries (Barrack et al., 2013). In addition to musculoskeletal injuries, another consequence of the female athlete triad is endothelial dysfunction that can lead to cardiovascular irregularities. Due to low estrogen levels brought about by amenorrhea, nitric oxide (NO) is not properly stimulated, hindering vasodilation. Additionally, anti-atherosclerotic properties normally facilitated by NO can be inhibited, leading to higher levels of triglycerides and high-density lipoproteins (Barrack et al., 2013).

Pharmacology

Pharmacological therapy for osteoporosis is mostly comprised of antiresorptives, and is designed to increase or stabilize BMD, or reduce bone loss. Antiresorptives include hormone replacement therapies, selective estrogen receptor modulators, bisphosphonates, and some antibodies. Anabolic drugs to stimulate osteoblastic bone formation are fairly new but offer a promising path to increase BMD. A list of common drugs and the side effects are in Table 24.2.

Table 24.2

Common drugs used for the treatment and prevention of osteoporosis

Antiresorptive	Preventive or Treatment	Effect	Side effects
Bisphosphonates	Prevention and treatment	Decrease bone resorption via osteoclast inhibition	GI disturbance Heartburn Headache
Receptor activator of nuclear factor kappa-B ligand (RANKL antibodies)	Treatment	Suppresses bone resorption via osteoclast inactivation	Increased risk for infection UTI
SERMS	Prevention and treatment	Interaction with bone's estrogen receptors Increase trabecular bone mass	Hot flashes Cramps Increased risk for blot clots
Calcitonin	Treatment	Increase osteoblast activity Inhibits osteoclast activity Reduces vertebral fracture risk	GI disturbance Headaches Flushing Allergic response
HRT	Prevention	Preserves BMD via a reduction in bone resorption Decreases fracture risk	Cancer Increased cardiovascular risk Stroke Blood clots
Anabolic agents	Treatment	Regulates blood calcium levels Osteoblast activation	Headache Nausea

Pavone et al., 2017; Sharp, 2018; Witzke, 2015

Nutrition

Nutrition is a vital for bone maintenance across the lifespan. Optimization can be achieved during childhood, adults can strive to maintain healthy bone, and seniors can prevent or treat osteoporosis (Mitchell et al., 2015). Calcium and Vitamin D are central to any nutrition plan for the prevention and treatment of osteoporosis (ACSM, 2018; Witzke, 2015). The dietary reference intake (DRI) for calcium is 200 mg/day for infants, an upper limit of 3000 mg/day for adolescents and pregnant women, and1200 mg/day females over age 50. Vitamin D is needed for calcium absorption and has a DRI of 400mg/day for infants, and an upper limit of 4000 mg/day for adolescents and pregnant women (ACSM, 2018).

Conversely, caffeine and alcohol may reduce bone strength by inhibiting calcium absorption, and Vitamin A can increase the risk of fractures from bone loss. Other important nutrients are in Table 24.3.

Table 24.3

Nutrients useful for the prevention and treatment of osteoporosis

Nutrient	Reasons/Benefits	Recommended amount	Source
Calcium	Comprises 50% of bone mass	Infants: 200-1000 mg/day Toddlers: 500-2500 mg/day Adolescents: 1100-3000 mg/day 50-70 years: 800-2500 mg/day > 70 years: 800-2000mg/day	Dairy Some varieties of fish Green, leafy vegetables
Vitamin D	Facilitates calcium absorption	Infants: 400-1000 mg/day Toddlers: 400-2500 mg/day Adolescents: 400-4000 mg/day 50-70 years: 400-4000 mg/day > 70 years: 400-4000/day	Sunshine Some fatty fish
Vitamin K	Activates some proteins May decrease risk of certain fractures	<18 years: 30-75 mcg/day > 18 years: 90-120 mcg/day	Dark green vegetables
Vitamin C	Helps the production of collagen	Adults: 75-90 mg/day	Citrus fruits Some berries Some peppers
Potassium	Helps with bone strength	Adults: 4.7 g/day	Fruits Vegetables Dairy Meat Nuts
Magnesium	Helps reduce calcium loss	Adults: 310-420 mg/day	Fruits Vegetables Nuts
Omega 3 fatty acids	Reduces systemic inflammation	Adults: 1-1.6 g/day	Fatty fish Nuts and seeds Some vegetables
Protein	Builds strong bones, particularly during childhood and adolescents	1-1.5 g/day per kg of bodyweight	Meat Dairy Eggs Beans

ACSM, 2018; Mitchell et al., 2015; Witzke, 2015

Exercise and Activity

Because bone formation occurs when people are young, it is important to optimize BMD during childhood and adolescence thorough loading activities. Weight bearing activities should be performed daily and moderate-to-vigorous activity has been shown to improve hip strength and bone structure (Fletcher, 2013). General bone-loading, even non-targeted activities including plyometrics, basketball, soccer, volleyball, gymnastics, and weight training can produce benefits, such as an increase in BMD into adulthood (Fletcher, 2013; Witzke, 2015).

Even though it is known anaerobic and aerobic exercise increase BMD and/or slow the progression of bone loss, there are no specific exercise guidelines for osteoporotic adults as recommendations should be based on the individual needs of each client (Chaconas, Olivencia, & Russ, 2013; Witzke, 2013). Because the skeletal response to activity is greatest at the site of maximum stress, exercises should target loading to at-risk bones. Exercise should be pain free, with a focus on weight bearing exercises and fall prevention (ACSM, 2018). Clients should be able to perform each movement with proper form, tissue health (bone, ligament, tendon, and muscle) needs to be considered during exercise selection, as does joint range of motion. Keep in mind any client who presents with osteoporosis needs a medical clearance to exercise and non-osteoporotic adults should follow the ACSM FITT guidelines for their specific situations.

Table 24.4 combines the exercise recommendations from numerous organizations and literature. Table 24.5 lists movements contraindicated for clients with osteoporosis.

Table 24.4

FITT recommendations for clients with osteopenia or osteoporosis

Exercise	Frequency	Intensity	Time	Type	Avoid
At-risk clients/osteopenia					
Aerobic	3-5 days/week	Light to moderate 40-70% HRR	30-60 minutes combined aerobic and resistance	Weight bearing • Walking • Running • Biking • Tennis • Stair stepper	• Any movement that causes pain • Explosive movements • Dynamic abdominal movements • Unsupported forward flexion • Excessive twisting, bending, or compression
Resistance Begin with 5-10 minutes of mild warm-up	2-3 days/week	60-80% 1RM 80-90% 1 RM	8-12 reps 5-6 reps 2-3 sets Rest as needed	• Modality based on assessment • Functional standing movements	
Neuromuscular	Daily			• Balance progression • Gait training	
Flexibility	5-7 days/week	Mild discomfort	3 stretches for each muscle group Hold for 15-30 seconds		
Clients with osteoporosis					
Aerobic	3-5 days/week	Light to moderate 40-60% HRR	30-60 minutes combined aerobic and resistance	No or low impact • Walking • Swimming • Stair climbing	
Resistance Begin with 5-10 minutes of mild warm-up	2-3 days/week	60-80% 1RM	8-12 reps	• Modality based on assessment • Bone loading movements • Functional standing movements	
Neuromuscular	Daily			• Balance progression • Gait training	
Flexibility	5-7 days/week	Mild discomfort	3 stretches for each muscle group Hold for 15-30 seconds		

ACSM, 2013; Sharp, 2018; Witzke, 2015

Table 24.5

Contraindicated movements for clients with osteoporosis

Exercise	Intention	Reason for concern
Yoga plough	Stretch low back	Compresses cervical spine
Neck circles/hyperextension	Relieves tension Stretches neck, traps, and shoulders	Compresses cervical nerve roots and arteries
Neck bridging	Strengthens neck	Compresses cervical discs
Straight-leg sit-up & Double leg lifts	Strengthens abdominals	Excessively stresses hips and low back
Standing toe touch	Stretches posterior chain	Forward flexion places stress on the low-back increasing risk for disc compression
Back hyperextension	Strengthens low back and hips	Increases risk for disc tissue damage
Hip twists	Stretch torso/strengthen abdominals	Increases risk for disc tissue damage, and hip capsular damage
Hurdler stretch Yoga lotus position	Stretch hamstring on the straight leg and quadriceps on the flexed leg	Places stress on the medial ligament of the flexed knee
Full squat	Strengthens lower body and core	Stresses ligaments and meniscus of the knee

ACSM, 2013; Sharp, 2018; Witzke, 2015

Discussion and application

1. Discuss the benefits of exercise and the guidelines for someone experiencing osteoporosis and/ or osteopenia.
2. Discuss the female triad and how it can effect BMD in males and females.

References

American College of Sports Medicine. (2018). *ACSM's resources for the exercise physiologist: A practical guide for the health fitness professional* (P. Magyari, R. Lite, M. W. Kilpatrick, & J. E. Schoffstall Eds. 2 ed.). Philadelphia, PA: Wolters Kluwer.

Bush, J. A. (2018). Female specific conditions in P.L. Jacobs (Ed) *NSCA's essentials of training special populations*. Champaign, IL: Human Kinetics.

Barrack, M. T., Ackerman, K. E., & Gibbs, J. C. (2013). Update on the female athlete triad. *Current Reviews in Musculoskeletal Medicine, 6*(2), 195-204. https://doi.org/10.1007/s12178-013-9168-9

Brandi, M.L. (2018). Genetics of osteoporosis. In: Lenzi A., Migliaccio S. (eds) *Multidisciplinary approach to osteoporosis*. Champaign, IL: Springer. https://doi.org/10.1007/978-3-319-75110-8_2

Chaconas, E. J., Olivencia, O., & Russ, B. S. (2013). Exercise interventions for the individual with osteoporosis. *Strength & Conditioning Journal, 35*(4), 49-55. http://dx.doi.org/10.1519/SSC.0b013e318291c6a5

Chesi, A., Wagley, Y., Johnson, M. E., Manduchi, E., Su, C., Lu, S.,...Grant, S. F. A. (2019). Genome-scale Capture C promoter interactions implicate effector genes at GWAS loci for bone mineral density. *Nature Communications, 10*(1), 1260. https://doi.org/10.1038/s41467-019-09302-x

Dempster, D. W. (2011). Osteoporosis and the burden of osteoporosis-related fractures. *The American Journal of Managed Care, 17*(6), s164-s169. Retrieved from http://www.ajmc.com/journals/supplement/2011/a357_may11/a357_11ma7__dempster_s164to169

Fletcher, J. A. (2013). Canadian academy of sport and exercise medicine position statement: Osteoporosis and exercise. *Clinical Journal of Sport Medicine, 23*(5), 333-338. https://doi.org/10.1097/JSM.0000000000000002

International Osteoporosis Foundation. (2017). Facts and statistics. Retrieved from https://www.iof-bonehealth.org/facts-statistics

Marini, F., Masi, L., Marcucci, G., Cianferotti, L., & Brandi, M.L. (2018). Genetics of osteoporosis. In: Lenzi A., Migliaccio S. (eds) *Multidisciplinary approach to osteoporosis*. Champaign, IL: Springer. https://doi.org/10.1007/978-3-319-75110-8_2

Mitchell, P. J., Cooper, C., Dawson-Hughes, B., Gordon, C. M., & Rizzoli, R. (2015). Life-course approach to nutrition. *Osteoporosis International, 26*(12), 2723-2742. https://doi.org/10.1007/s00198-015-3288-6

National Institutes of Health. (2018). Osteoporosis. Retrieved from https://report.nih.gov/NIHfactsheets/ViewFactSheet.aspx?csid=56&key=O

National Osteoporosis Foundation. (2014). 54 million Americans affected by osteoporosis and low bone mass: NOF releases updated data detailing the prevalence of osteoporosis and low bone mass in the U.S. Retrieved from https://www.nof.org/news/54-million-americans-affected-by-osteoporosis-and-low-bone-mass/

National Human Genome Research Institute. (2018). What is the human genome project? Retrieved from https://www.genome.gov/human-genome-project/What.

Pavone, V., Testa, G., Giardina, S. M. C., Vescio, A., Restivo, D. A., & Sessa, G. (2017). Pharmacological therapy of osteoporosis: A systematic current review of literature. *Frontiers in Pharmacology, 8*, 803. https://doi.org/10.3389/fphar.2017.00803

Sharp, C. (2018). Musculoskeletal conditions and disorders in P.L. Jacobs (Ed*) NSCA's essentials of training special populations*. Champaign, IL: Human Kinetics

Sozen, T., Ozisik, L., & Basaran, N. C. (2017). An overview and management of osteoporosis. *European Journal of Rheumatology, 4*(1), 46-56. https://doi.org/10.5152/eurjrheum.2016.048

Witzke, K. A. (2015). Osteoporosis and osteopenia in J.S. Skinner, C.X. Bryant, S. Merrill, & D.J. Green (Eds), *American Council on Exercise medical exercise specialist manual.* San Diego, CA: American Council on Exercise.

CHAPTER 25
BUSINESS CONSIDERATIONS

By the end of this chapter you will understand:

- Types of business entities
- HIPAA regulations
- Social media
- SOAP notes
- Ethical considerations

Business Entities

Not everyone will open their own business, but health and fitness professionals need to understand the implications of business, ethics, and legal matters, particularly as we interact with other healthcare providers. For fitness professionals who wish to open their own business, a good place to start is by knowing the types of business entities. The type of structure will determine the taxes that need to be filed and liability ramifications (U.S. Small Business Administration [SBA], n.d.).

A sole proprietorship is easy to form but does not create a separate business entity, and therefore, does not protect an owner against liability claims because the business and the owner are considered the same. In other words, all business assets are considered personal assets and an owner can be held liable for any claims made against the business. This is type of entity is appropriate for very low-risk businesses or if a business is just starting and wants to demonstrate a concept.

A limited liability company (LLC) provides personal protection from claims made against a company. It is easy to form, can be created by an individual or a group, and allows profits and losses from a company to be passed through to the personal taxes of the members without the need to file separate corporate taxes. However, if a member leaves, the LLC may need to be dissolved and a new LLC may need to be formed. An LLC is good option for a business that involves some risk (such as a fitness studio), the owner(s) have some assets to be protected, and the corporate tax is too high.

A partnership is a cross between a LLC and a sole proprietorship. There are two partnerships types. A Limited Partnership (LP) has one general partner who takes on all of the liability, while a Limited Liability Partnership (LLP) protects each partner from the debts of the partnership and from each of the other partners.

A C Corp is a separate entity from the owners and provides legal protection for an owner's personal assets. Corporations pay taxes on their profits at the corporate tax rate, and again on the distribution of dividends. Funds can be raised through the sale of corporate stock and owners can leave by simply selling their stock. The cost to start a corporation is high and there is extensive legal paperwork.

An S Corp is similar to a C Corp, except the profits and losses are passed through to an owner's personal taxes. Not all states recognize or allow S Corps, but for States that do, there is a limit of 100 shareholders and all shareholders must be citizens of the United States.

There are other forms of corporations such as B Corps (benefit corp), closed corporations, non-profits, and cooperatives. A list of the salient points of each is in Table 25.1 (SBA, n.d.).

Table 25.1

Business structures in the United States

Business structure	Ownership	Liability	Taxes
Sole proprietorship	One person	Unlimited personal liability	Personal tax only
Partnerships	Two or more people	Unlimited personal liability unless structured as a limited partnership	Self-employment tax (except for limited partners) Personal tax
Limited liability company (LLC)	One or more people	Owners are not personally liable	Self-employment tax Personal tax or corporate tax
Corporation—C corp	One or more people	Owners are not personally liable	Corporate tax
Corporation—S corp	One or more people, but no more than 100, and all must be U.S. citizens	Owners are not personally liable	Personal tax
Corporation—B corp	One or more people	Owners are not personally liable	Corporate tax
Corporation—Nonprofit	One or more people	Owners are not personally liable	Tax-exempt, but corporate profits can't be distributed

SBA, n.d.

The Health Insurance Portability and Accountability Act

The Health Insurance Portability and Accountability Act (HIPAA), enacted in 1996, provides continuous health insurance coverage, standardized the electronic transmission of transactions, and eliminated waste (Rouse, Biscobing, & Sutner, n.d.). Although HIPAA contains five sections, a CXS is most concerned with part of section 2 that includes the Standards for Privacy of Individually Identifiable Health Information, or the HIPAA Privacy Rule. The HIPAA Privacy Rule established laws and safeguards to protect the privacy of personal, identifiable health information. While most health clubs and personal trainers do not have to adhere to HIPAA regulations, in some instances, if CXSs collaborate with physicians, registered dieticians, physical therapists, or massage therapists they may have to adhere to HIPAA regulations (Larcom, 2018). A CXS who collaborates with a clinician and shares client information electronically must follow HIPAA regulations. Also, if any licensed clinician (physician, physician assistant, physical therapist, chiropractor, massage therapist. etc.) a CXS shares information with is considered covered under the HIPAA laws, a CXS must also comply (Larcom, 2018). Regardless, most clients appreciate the professionalism associated with the healthcare community and expect a degree of confidentiality. Some guidelines to consider under HIPAA are (U.S. Department of Health and Human Services, 2013):

- **Who/What is covered?**
    - o Health Plans—Individual and group plans that provide or pay the cost of medical care are covered entities.
    - o Health Care Providers and Providers of Services—Every health care provider and provider of medical or health services regardless of size, who electronically transmits health information in connection with certain transactions, is a covered entity. Transactions can include shared databases, emailed personal information, electronic billing, etc.
    - o Business Associates—A person or organization, other than a member of a covered entity's workforce, who performs certain functions or activities on behalf of, or provides certain services to, a covered entity that involves the use or disclosure of individually identifiable health information.
- **What information is protected?**
    - o The Privacy Rule protects all individually identifiable health information (defined as demographic information, past, present or future physical or mental health or condition, or the type of care provided or planned) held or transmitted by a covered entity or its business associate, in any form or media, whether electronic, paper, or oral.
    - o Other individually identifiable health information includes many common identifiers such as name, address, birth date, or social security number.
- **De-Identified health information**
    - o There are no restrictions on the use or disclosure of de-identified health information. De-identified health information neither identifies nor provides a reasonable basis to identify an individual.

- **Release of information**
  - Information may be released with a client's consent.
  - The authorization must include:
    - The name of the person or entity releasing the information.
    - The name of the person or entity to whom the information is being released.
    - A description of the information to be used or disclosed.
    - How the information will be used.
    - An expiration date or event.
    - An explanation of a patient's right to revoke the authorization needs to be included.
    - No blank spaces to be filled out by the provider can be used.
    - The authorization form must be in plain language.
    - The client's signature and date.
    - A copy must be provided to the patient.

Ensuring client confidentiality displays discretion and professionalism. Confidentiality also minimizes the risk of ethical misconduct or legal action. All client information should be kept in a locked cabinet or a password-protected computer, file, or cloud drive (Coors, 2015). Any discussion regarding clients, whether in person or electronically should be held in a private space, and information should only be shared with the client and any clinical professional from whom a release has been obtained.

Social Media

Social media has become both a tool and a hindrance for health professionals. Social media includes social networking, blogs, file sharing cloud drives, and print, photograph, or video web publishing. Posting pictures and videos of clients, workouts, and progress has become standard marketing practice. A social networking or blog post can reach millions of viewers and potential clients instantly, shared documents can be accessed by numerous users from anywhere in the world and before and after pictures, or workout videos can bolster engagement. However, for all the positive aspects of social media, there are risks, particularly when personal and professional accounts are mixed (Scruth, Pugh, Adams, & Foss-Durant, 2015).

One risk of using social media is the violation of HIPAA. Without prior consent, the use of any personal information to include, name, photographic or video likeness, or personal description can be considered a HIPAA violation. Documents shared via a cloud drive can allow for access and dissemination of personal information worldwide, and a blog post with written, personal descriptors may provide enough information to identify someone.

Another risk of social media is the instant scrutiny of controversial opinions, behaviors, or shared content. Political points of view are often considered contentious and may lead to vile debate. Behaviors that may be in conflict with the standards of a health and fitness professional, such as drinking alcohol, smoking, or indulging in unhealthy nutritional habits, may suggest a *do as I say, not as I do* attitude, and alienate potential clients and colleagues. Content shared from other sources such as memes or gifs may be considered amusing to some, but others may find it inappropriate. When entering a virtual atmosphere, keep in mind professional standards cannot be negated, information presented should be unbiased and evidence based, and unsubstantiated assertions should never be made. Most importantly, do not record, in any form (written, video, photographic) anything you do not want made public or presented in a court of law.

SOAP Notes

A detailed, confidential file should be maintained on each client. The file should include a waiver, assessment information, workout records, a medical release when needed, a signed PAR-Q or Physical Activity Risk Stratification form, and any other pertinent information. In the event information needs to be shared with other clinical professionals, SOAP notes should be used to convey client information in a concise format. SOAP stands for subjective, objective, assessment, and plan (Blue Cross Blue Shield of Alabama, n.d.; Coors, 2015; The CHP Group. n.d.). The specific information for each section is listed below.

- Subjective—In a client's own words, what is the reason for the visit? In follow-up notes, any change of the original reason for the visit should be noted.
- Objective—What are the signs and symptoms that can be measured such as pain, movement dysfunction, vital signs, and anthropometric measurements?
- Assessment—What are the results of measurements taken and assessments performed? Any history relevant to the present condition should be mentioned. For example, if the client sprained an ankle 3 months ago, and has asymmetric weight shifting while performing a squat assessment, it is relevant and should be noted. Remember this is not a diagnosis, but a clear, concise statement of the findings while staying within the scope of practice.
- Plan—What course of action is suggested? Is the plan in the scope of practice of a fitness professional or does the client need to be referred to a clinical provider? The plan should answer the following questions and should be updated as the initial plan progresses:
    - What is being done for a client and why?
    - What is a client to do or not do and why?
    - When will a client return and why?

In addition to the actual SOAP part of the document, the date, a client's name, date of birth, address, and contact information should be included. It may also be prudent to include information regarding adherence to the plan, missed appointments, and any other updates the provider thinks are important. A copy of an example SOAP note template can be found in Appendix D.

Ethical Considerations

Every aspect of ethics should reinforce the responsibility of a CXS to provide safe, effective instruction within the scope of practice and is limited to the knowledge, skills, and abilities of a CXS. Every certifying organization has a code of ethics designed to provide guidance and set common ethical standards that promote uniform behavior. The following is a compilation of standards from a number of fitness organizations (American College of Sports Medicine, 2005; American Council on Exercise, n.d.; National Academy of Sports Medicine, n.d.):

- Provide safe and effective instruction that is consistent with evidence-based science and medicine.
- Provide and maintain an environment to ensure client safety.
- Behave in a manner that merits the respect of clients, the public, and other colleagues.
- Treat every colleague and client equally with the utmost respect and dignity.
- Do not make false or derogatory assumptions concerning the practices of colleagues and clients.
- Use appropriate professional communication in all verbal, non-verbal, and written transactions.
- Establish and maintain clear professional boundaries.
- Maintain a level of personal hygiene appropriate for a health and fitness setting.
- Wear clothing that is clean, modest, and professional.
- Remain in good standing and maintain certification status by acquiring all necessary continuing education requirements.
- Stay up to date on the latest health and fitness research and understand its practical application.
- Maintain CPR certification and knowledge of first-aid services.
- Honestly and truthfully represent all professional qualifications and affiliations, and the limitations of expertise.
- Provide services consistent with the boundaries of knowledge, skills, and abilities, and do not provide services limited by state law to provision by another health care professional only.
- Refer a client to the appropriate medical practitioner when conditions fall outside the scope of practice of a CXS.
- Respect the confidentiality of all clients, colleagues, and health professionals, and safeguard confidences within the boundaries of the law.
- Maintain adequate and truthful progress notes for each client.
- Comply with all legal requirements in the applicable jurisdiction.
- Maintain adequate liability insurance.
- Accurately and truthfully inform the public of services rendered and qualifications to render such services.
- Maintain accurate financial, contract, appointment, and tax records.
- Comply with all applicable business, employment, and intellectual property laws.

Discussion and application

1. What are SOAP notes? Write a SOAP note for a current client.
2. Discuss the origin, the benefits, and the downside of HIPAA.

References

American College of Sports Medicine. (2005). Code of ethics for ACSM certified and registered professionals. Retrieved from http://www.kines.umich.edu/sites/default/files/eth_acsm_code_of_ethics.pdf

American Council on Exercise. (n.d.). Code of ethics. Retrieved from https://acewebcontent.azureedge.net/assets/certification/pdfs/CodeofEthics.pdf

Blue Cross Blue Shield of Alabama. (n.d.). Medical documentation tips: The SOAP note. Retrieved from https://providers.bcbsal.org/portal/documents/10226/306297/Medical+Documentation+Tips/98b50e9d-816d-464d-a0a7-9fbe11d5438c?version=1.0

Coors, L. (2015). Professional relationships and business strategies in J.S. Skinner, C.X. Bryant, S. Merrill, & D.J. Green (Eds), *American Council on Exercise medical exercise specialist manual.* San Diego, CA: American Council on Exercise

Larcom, A. B. (2018). Does your health club need to comply with HIPAA? Retrieved from https://www.ihrsa.org/improve-your-club/does-your-health-club-need-to-comply-with-hipaa/#

National Academy of Sports Medicine. (n.d.). NASM code of professional conduct. Retrieved from https://www.nasm.org/docs/default-source/PDF/nasm-code-of-professional-conduct.pdf?sfvrsn=2

Rouse, M., Biscobing, J., & Sutner, S. (n.d.). HIPAA (Health Insurance Portability and Accountability Act). Retrieved from https://searchhealthit.techtarget.com/definition/HIPAA

Scruth, E. A., Pugh, D. M., Adams, C. L., & Foss-Durant, A. M. (2015). Electronic and social media: The legal and ethical issues for healthcare. *Clinical Nurse Specialist, 29*(1), 8-11. https://doi.org/10.1097/NUR.0000000000000089

The CHP Group. (n.d.) Best practices in clinical record keeping: SOAP notes. Retrieved from http://www.chpgroup.com/images/Documents/helper%20packet/BestPracticesSOAP.pdf

U.S. Small Business Administration. (n.d.). Choose a business structure. Retrieved from https://www.sba.gov/business-guide/launch-your-business/choose-business-structure

U.S. Department of Health and Human Services. (2013). Summary of the HIPAA Privacy Rule. Retrieved from https://www.hhs.gov/hipaa/for-professionals/privacy/laws-regulations/index.html

APPENDICES

Appendix A—Sample Physical Activity Risk Stratification form

Name____ Date______________________

Name of physician________________________________ Number_______________________

Based on the information below does the client need to obtain a medical clearance prior to exercise? YES NO

Do you participate in regular exercise (structured physical activity for at least 30 minutes 3x/week for the last 3 months)	Yes	No	Unknown
If yes at what level:			
• Light – Slight increase in HR and breathing (30-40HRR; 2-3 METS; RPE 9-11)			
• Moderate – Noticeable increase in HR and breathing (40-60 HRR; 3-6 METS; RPE 12-13)			
• Vigorous – Substantial increase in HR and breathing (60-90 HRR; 6-8 METS; RPE 14-17)			
Do you have cardiovascular disease including, but not limited to coronary heart disease, hypertension, arrhythmia, or peripheral artery disease?			
Do you currently have, or have you ever had a heart attack (myocardial infarction), stroke, congestive heart failure, or congenital heart disease?			
Do you have any type of diabetes?			
Do you have any of the following? (Three or more indicate metabolic syndrome, and an increased risk for metabolic or cardiovascular disease)			
• Abdominal obesity as indicated by a waist circumference of ≥40" for men or ≥35" for women			
• Triglyceride levels of ≥ 150 mg/dl			
• HDL levels of <40 mg/dl for men and <50 mg/dl for women			
• Blood pressure ≥ 130/85 mm/Hg			
• Fasting glucose level of ≥100 mg/dl			
At rest, or during activity do you, or have you in the past 12 months, experienced any of the following:			
• Pain or discomfort in the chest, neck, jaw, arms, or other areas that may result from ischemia			
• Shortness of breath at rest or during mild exertion, or orthopnea or paroxysmal nocturnal dyspnea			
• Dizziness or syncope			
• Ankle edema			
• Palpitations or tachycardia, or a racing, pounding, or fluttering heart			
• Intermittent claudication or leg pain			
• Heart murmur			
• Unusual fatigue or shortness of breath while performing usual activity			
Has your doctor ever said that you should only do medically supervised physical activity?			
Have you had a physical in the last12 months?			

Use the answers from the questionnaire, and follow the chart below to determine the need for a medical clearance to begin exercise, and at what intensity.

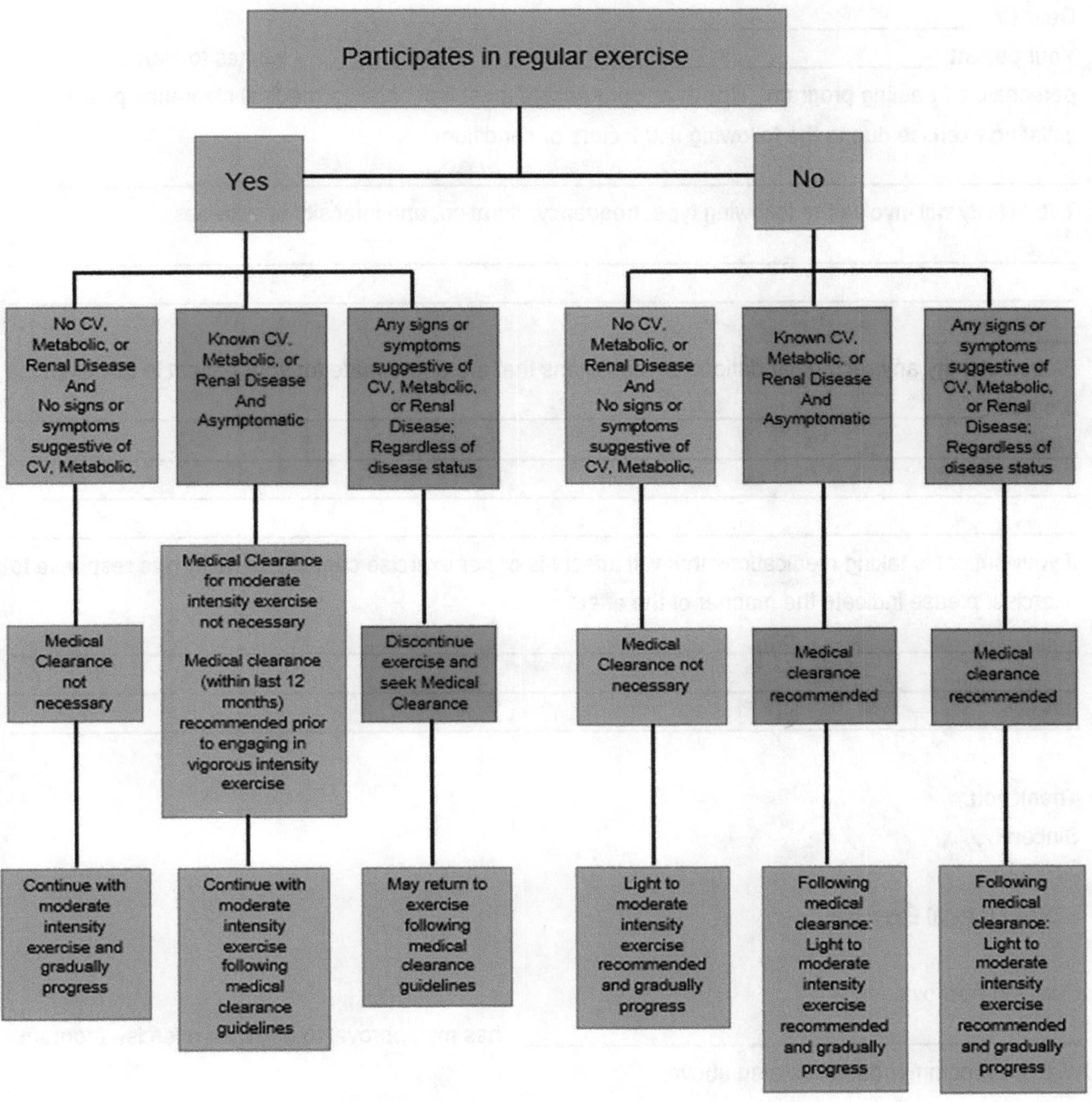

Appendix B—Sample Medical Clearance form

Date ____________________

Dear Dr: ________________________

Your patient, ____, wishes to start a personalized training program. However, your patient must first obtain a medical clearance prior to initiating exercise due to the following risk factors or conditions:

____

The activity will involve the following type, frequency, duration, and intensity of activities:

____

____

____

Please identify any recommendations or restrictions that are appropriate for your patient in this exercise program:____

____

____

____

If your patient is taking medications that will affect his or her exercise capacity or heart-rate response to exercise, please indicate the manner of the effect:

____

____

____

Thank you.

Sincerely,

NOVA Medical Exercise

Clinician Approval:

____ has my approval to begin an exercise program with the recommendations stated above.

____

Signature Date

Appendix C—YMCA Bench Step Assessment for Cardiovascular Fitness

Testing for cardiovascular fitness can be costly, time consuming, and also require elaborate equipment. The YMCA Step Test is easy to implement in almost any setting. The YMCA 3-minute Bench Step Test is based on how quickly your heart rate recovers following a short bout of exercise.

Below are the essentials to perform the test on your own

- 12-inch tall step, bench, or box (as close to 12 inches as you can find)
- Stopwatch, timer, or clock with a secondhand
- Metronome (there are a number of free apps available for Android and IOS)
- Heart rate monitor (optional)
- Partner to assist with cadence and form (optional)

Procedures

1. Set the metronome to 96 beats per minute and turn the volume up loud enough that you can hear each beat.
2. Stand facing your step.
3. When ready to begin start the stopwatch or timer and begin stepping on and off the step to the metronome beat following a cadence of up, up, down, down.
4. Continue for 3 minutes.
5. As soon as you reach 3 minutes, stop immediately and sit down on your step.
6. Perform a manual pulse reading and count the number of beats for an entire **60 seconds.** If wearing a heart rate monitor record your heart rate 1 minute from when you sit down.
7. Record your pulse when you have reached 1 minute and then locate your score on the rating scale below.

YMCA Step Test Ratings						
Age	**18-25**	**26-35**	**36-45**	**46-55**	**56-65**	**65+**
Women						
Excellent	52-81	58-80	51-84	63-91	60-92	70-92
Good	85-93	85-92	89-96	95-101	97-103	96-101
Above Average	96-102	95-101	100-104	104-110	106-111	104-111
Average	104-110	104-110	107-112	113-118	113-118	116-121
Below Average	113-120	113-119	115-120	120-124	119-127	123-126
Poor	122-131	122-129	124-132	126-132	129-135	128-133
Very Poor	135-169	134-171	137-169	137-171	141-174	135-155
Men						
Excellent	50-76	51-76	49-76	56-82	60-77	59-81
Good	79-84	79-85	80-88	87-93	86-94	87-92
Above Average	88-93	88-94	92-88	95-101	97-100	94-102
Average	95-100	96-102	100-105	103-111	103-109	104-110
Below Average	102-107	104-110	108-113	113-119	111-117	114-118
Poor	111-119	114-121	116-124	121-126	119-128	121-126
Very Poor	124-157	126-161	130-163	131-159	131-154	130-151

Appendix D—Sample SOAP Notes form

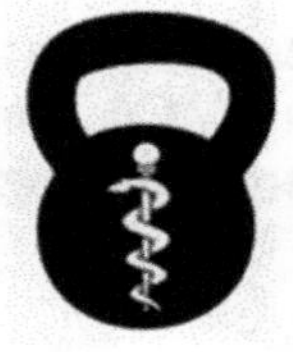

NOVA Medical Exercise

Connecting education, medicine, and fitness

SOAP Notes for:
Client Name ______________________ DOB ______________

Address ______________________ Phone ______________

Physician ______________________ Phone ______________

Subjective:

____
____
____
____

Objective:

____
____
____
____

Assessment:

____
____
____
____

Plan:

____
____
____
____

Additional Notes:

1. ______________________
2. ______________________
3. ______________________
4. ______________________
5. ______________________

Completed By ______________________ Date of contact______________

AUTHOR BIO

For over 20 years Dr. Dan Mikeska has been the owner of **NOVA Medical Exercise** – a fitness studio dedicated to helping clients control, minimize, and even overcome chronic disease through fitness. He's also the creator of the **Medical Exercise Academy** which specializes in educating health and fitness professionals on the effects of exercise on chronic disease. He has a master's degree in Human Movement and a doctorate in Health Science, and teaches graduate kinesiology classes for A. T. Still University.

Dr. Mikeska holds numerous certifications from the National Academy of Sports Medicine, the American Council on Exercise, the Cancer Exercise Training Institute, and Exercise is Medicine. He became interested in fitness as a means to improve in martial arts, and he holds belts or instructor ranks in Jeet Kune Do Concepts, Combat Submission Wrestling, American Sport Karate, and is a Universal and United States Martial Arts Hall of Fame inductee. He is on the Medical Exercise Review Board for the Cancer Exercise Training Institute as well as the Industry Advisory Council for American Public University System's Sports and Health Science program.

As the author of numerous published articles on metabolic conditioning programs for martial artists, the scope of practice for fitness trainers, and the state of online education and medical exercise, he's recognized as one of the top educators on fitness and chronic disease. He and his wife live in Northern Virginia, and he can be reached at www.MedEx.fit.

Printed in the USA
CPSIA information can be obtained
at www.ICGtesting.com
LVHW080441281023
762038LV00004B/4